Does My Child Need a Therapist?

Colleen Alexander-Roberts
and
Mark Snyder, M.D.

TAYLOR PUBLISHING COMPANY
Dallas, Texas

For my children, Christopher and Blake Roberts;
and my brothers, Mark and Matthew.
—Colleen

In loving memory of my parents, Larry and Bernice Snyder.
You are missed and loved.
I finally "get it."
—Mark

Published by Taylor Publishing Company
1550 West Mockingbird Lane
Dallas, Texas 75235

The information contained in this book is not intended to serve as a replacement for
professional medical or legal advice or professional psychological counseling. Any
use of the information in this book is at the reader's discretion. The author and
publisher specifically disclaim any and all liability arising directly or indirectly
from the use or application of any information contained in this book. The
appropriate professional should be consulted regarding specific conditions.

Library of Congress Cataloging-in-Publication Data

Alexander-Roberts, Colleen.
    Does my child need a therapist? / Colleen Alexander-Roberts and
Mark Snyder.
        p.   cm.
    Includes bibliographical references and index.
    ISBN 0-87833-942-6
    1. Child psychiatry—Popular works. 2. Emotional problems of children.
I. Snyder, Mark (Mark T.) II. Title.
RJ499.34.A44   1997
618.92'89—dc21   96-29588
                                                                CIP

Printed in the United States of America

10   9   8   7   6   5   4   3   2   1

CONTENTS

Appendices

Acknowledgments

Colleen Alexander-Roberts

A very special thank you to Louis B. Cady, M.D., a board-certified child and adolescent psychiatrist, writer, and lecturer, in Evansville, Indiana. You came through again for me, Louis, with your support, insight, and well-written foreword! It's your turn next, friend.

Many thanks also to the members of the ADD forum on CompuServe, particularly Nancylynn Lockman and Dana Weldon for sharing their ideas, thoughts, disappointments, and successes, and to all of my other friends on CompuServe and America Online who shared their positive and negative stories about therapy. To Daphne Kent of CompuServe, who helps me more than she ever realizes. Thanks, Daphne, for everything.

Thanks also to my editor, Macy Jaggers, for her ideas and suggestions; Jason Rath, assistant editor, for his patience and marvelous editing; and the rest of the Taylor staff for supporting this project from its inception.

My gratitude to two wonderful, dear friends, Christine Adamec and Judith Gilbert, who have stood by me through thick and thin with their love and support through the years, but especially over the past year when I needed them the most.

And to my best friend, Mark Snyder, M.D., a special thank you for agreeing to write this book with me. Your support, understanding, encouragement, and belief in me mean more than you'll ever realize. You're a terrific writer, copartner, and wonderful friend of children.

I thank my wonderful parents, Joanne and Stan, for their encouragement, love, and support; and my brothers, Mark and Matt, for their love, numerous laughs, and late-night phone calls. My two wonderful sons, Christopher and Blake, have always been a major source of inspiration. Together we've traveled a long road paved with lots of happiness and more than a bit of sadness, but now there's peace in the home, the moon is full, and the forecast is sunny and bright. We're never alone as long as we have each other. I love you both.

Colleen Alexander-Roberts

Mark T. Snyder, M.D.

Many people helped prepare me, over the years, for my part in writing this book—family, friends, teachers, patients. I've been very fortunate to have had a number of outstanding members of the profession befriend and guide me in my professional and personal development and become lifelong friends as well.

Two such sources of inspiration generously became mentors of mine. To Peter Weiser, M.D., and Howard Wulsin, M.D., two fine psychiatrists, I give my everlasting appreciation and admiration. They modeled for me the highest standards of professional concern, empathy, and genuine regard for the inherent value of those who consult us, our patients.

Moran Menendez, M.D., a teacher, friend, and confidant, helped so much in developing my insight into the minds of our patients. His wry wit, dry humor, and New York accent (in Phoenix, Arizona!) often hid his warmth and sensitivity, protecting with a superficial gruffness the warmth of a teddy bear, the razor sharpness of a Socratic scholar.

A cyberfriend and colleague, Louis B. Cady, M.D., always willing to share his considerable expertise despite his busy schedule, took the time to review and comment on our manuscript. Thanks for the wonderful foreword, Louis!

My coauthor, Colleen Alexander-Roberts, who tolerated my stumbling efforts to match her literary acumen, is also the best mother I've ever been fortunate enough to meet. She has used her heart as a guide and her great intellect to turn her love for her children into "right action," and I commend her to you as someone worth listening to. Against tremendous odds and active interference, she's fought for greater understanding of the problems of children everywhere. Seeing the pain on the faces of both her boys as they struggled with their own difficulties and uncertainties, she became their champion. Her books are her personal contribution to the hope of better days for all troubled children.

Thanks to our editor, Macy Jaggers, and Jason Rath, our assistant editor. Jason, you needed the patience of Job and the wisdom of Solomon in editing my part of our book. You did a great job, Jason. Thanks for being gentle!

Most importantly, I thank my patients for the privilege of caring for them. Being allowed to share in their pain and sorrows as well as the joys and successes they experience as they grow, has been the greatest and most rewarding part of my continuing medical education. To those I've known and those I've yet to meet, thank you.

And thank you, Bernice; thank you, Larry. Your hard work and struggle may have finally borne fruit. Thanks for not giving up. You did a better job than you lived to see, but, being parents, you knew that, didn't you?

Mark Snyder, M.D.

Foreword

"Does my child need a therapist?" is not only the title for this book but also a question that I am frequently called upon to answer in the course of my practice of child, adolescent, and adult psychiatry. The book that you are holding in your hands will not only assist you in answering that question definitely and confidently but will also provide you with much more.

Ms. Alexander-Roberts and Dr. Snyder, two wonderful, witty, and thoroughly enjoyable people, have crafted a most unusual book. The mere elucidation of the answer to the question of whether or not therapy is indicated for a young person is, within the skills of a competent and skilled mental health professional, frequently not all that difficult. Nor is it especially difficult to engage a child in therapy. Most children, except the most profoundly disturbed, can be helped if approached empathetically and in a caring, nonthreatening manner by a good therapist. Indeed, in my experience, most children actually seem to blossom in a wholesome therapeutic relationship and ultimately find the experience quite satisfying—even if at the conclusion they are still too young to articulate what has just transpired and why they are feeling better. They just know they *are* and that they, Mommy, and Daddy all seem to be getting along much better.

Actually, the most fundamental and vexing issue encountered in getting children the help they need involves, strangely enough, the parents. Parents, after all, are real people too! They are typically alarmed at the strange turn of events that their child's life has taken. Often, they are covertly worried that they might have "done something wrong" in their parenting. Frequently, they are confronting an issue in their child that is simply so incredibly out of the context of their normal day-to-day existence that they haven't a clue as to what might have occurred or even who to ask!

It is here that Ms. Alexander-Roberts and Dr. Snyder's book is of such benefit. Although written for the layperson, it is exhaustively detailed, not "dumbed down," and basically amounts to a crash course in the possible psychological difficulties that your child could be experiencing. It is well laid out, highly structured, and not only can be read cover to cover but also can be bored into at various chapter levels for quick and specific answers to urgent questions.

Does My Child Need a Therapist? begins with the exploration of parents' fears and anxieties when it appears that their child needs help; it cautions against getting overly concerned and "jumping the gun" by rushing in to professionally evaluate what might be a relatively benign fluctuation in a child's functioning. Good communication with the child is emphasized here, as it is in the rest of this book. Most importantly, however, this section sets the stage for some reflection on the part of the parents about how their *own* childhood might have impacted their parenting style and how that could be affecting their relationship with their child. That is also how the book ends: with a gentle invitation for the family to get involved, participate in the therapy, and learn how all members of the family can contribute to getting the identified patient—a child, in this case—well! How wonderful. This book is about the holistic practice of psychiatry and psychology—not about pushing pills or engaging in a lengthy and unproductive course of therapy but about marshaling a family's resources to work on the problem together.

To do that, of course, some fundamental knowledge is required. That breadth of knowledge is presented in abundance in this volume, encompassing every common and even uncommon mental disorder of childhood and adolescence. Furthermore, the potential for a disproportionate emotional response to what might actually be relatively minor "psychological difficulties" is sensitively addressed. This explication serves not only to sketch in the themes that should be explored in therapy, but also to reassure the parents that they didn't "cause all the problems." Children, in their own marvelous creative mental playgrounds, can conjure up fairy godmothers and wonderful magic spells as well as self-imposed curses and mental hauntings designed, engineered, and built by their own as yet imperfect understanding of the world and their role in it.

After my detailed reading of this book, I would offer the following "road map" to the general reader. You will not only be able to definitively answer the question of whether or not therapy is indicated, but you will also know, within a reasonable margin of certainty, the answers to these questions:

- Just what is most likely wrong with my child? Is it a purely "biological" or inherited difficulty? Did I unknowingly do something to exacerbate it?

- Who should I get to treat my child? Where do I find her?

- What are the various forms of treatment available? Should psychiatric medications be used? Are they harmful? Addictive? Dangerous?

- How do I know if the therapy is progressing well? What should I be told by the therapist? What do I have a right to be told?

- In what kinds of settings should therapy, or even more aggressive treatment programs like "inpatient treatment," be conducted?

- What can we as a family do to help?

Parents who finish this book will have undergone a profound change. They will have far more data at their fingertips than many medical professionals. They will at least have a clue as to where and in what domain lie the problems that their child is experiencing. They will have the answers to all of the questions listed above. In short, parents will be well versed, empowered, and emboldened to find and secure the best therapy required to quickly begin dealing with the problems in their child's life that brought them to this book and the exploration of psychotherapy in the first place. They will be full partners with the treating physician, psychologist, or therapist in getting their loved one better as soon as possible.

The result of that intellectual change, and the ultimate result of this book, is nothing short of profound. In terms of getting the psychological help that a child needs, this intellectual and cognitive change parallels perfectly the goal of the healing arts: to restore the sick to health, and in the case of psychological illness, to restore the suffering soul's ability to reclaim the capacity to experience love, joy, happiness, and the incredible adventure of existence.

Louis B. Cady, M.D.
Evansville, Indiana

PART I

When Something Doesn't Seem Quite Right: Facing Childhood Problems

ONE

You're Not Alone

Most parents have concerns about their children. We worry about such things as our children's health, behavior, and whether they are eating and sleeping appropriately for their age. We also worry about their education and how they are developing compared to other children the same age. Our concerns are normal because we love our children. Most often, our concerns resolve on their own as our children continue to grow and flourish.

Sometimes, however, our concerns are well founded and may escalate to genuine alarm. Maybe you've witnessed disturbing problems in your child that you don't understand, like aggressive or bizarre behaviors or perhaps an unusual amount of crying over several weeks. Maybe you've learned that your child has been skipping school or is flunking in school despite her demonstrated capability. Or maybe a neighbor told you that your son tossed a rock through his window, and your son responded only by saying, "I don't know why I did it!" Or you may have concerns like the parents in the following stories.

Anxious and concerned about appearing foolish and overly protective, Susan stammered slightly as she prepared to talk about her seven-year-old son, Jason, with the pediatrician.

"Doctor, I'm concerned," she began. "Jason's second-grade teacher, Mrs. Hewlett, really likes him, says that she thinks he's very creative and bright. . . . " Tears started to fill her eyes as she continued. "But she also says that he seems to have trouble paying attention during class; it's as if he's in another world. But when he's not staring, he's often disruptive in class. She says he has no friends because he is so bossy, and emotionally she thinks he has some problems. His grades are falling . . . and I don't know what to do. I've tried talking with him, but it's as if he doesn't care."

Phylis, not sure who to discuss Jeanie's eating problem with, looked up as Dr. Compton, her internist, entered the office and greeted her warmly. Successful with her own advertising agency, Phylis was usually full of confidence, bright, and bubbly. Today, however, she felt a knot in the pit of her stomach that had ached since she first realized that her fifteen-year-old daughter, Jeanie, always thin as a rail, was binging on junk food, then making herself vomit. Phylis had heard of it, of course; it was called bulimia. But wasn't bulimia a . . . mental disorder? The thought of her precious Jeanie having a mental problem frightened her. She also felt vaguely guilty; hadn't she always told Jeanie to clean her plate? Maybe Phylis was the cause of this all. Dr. Compton would know what to do, though, wouldn't he?

"A child psychiatrist! For Ryan?" Steve had almost shouted the words, feeling hurt and angry. His wife of fifteen years, Lois, looked at him with fear in her eyes, her hands nervously fidgeting in her lap. Dr. Stack, a pediatrician, had seen "the look" before. Parents with a troubled child, on first hearing her recommendation that they take their child to see Dr. Jenkins, her favorite child psychiatrist, always had a troubled look: fear mixed with disbelief, anxiety laced with guilt, that they'd somehow failed as parents.

You're Not Alone

If you've ever felt like any of these parents, you're far from alone. Of the seventy million or so children up to age eighteen, perhaps as many as one-third, or more than twenty-three million, have had, now have, or will have an emotional disorder, developmental disorder, or disruptive behavior disorder that warrants psychological or psychiatric intervention. Sadly, according to a senior child psychiatrist at the National Institute of Mental Health (NIMH), estimates are that from two-thirds to as many as four-fifths of such youngsters will not receive the care and attention they deserve.

Children who have undiagnosed and untreated emotional, developmental, or behavioral disorders pay a high price, as do their families. Undiagnosed and untreated disorders interfere with the child's normal development, which then affects the entire course of the child's life. Intervention with therapy and sometimes with medication during childhood can prevent significant harm to the child and reduce or even prevent distress and upset in the child's adolescent and adult years.

Making Sense of Your Child's Problems

Recognizing the difference between normal, age-appropriate behavior and behavior that is problematic is not always easy. Because children's behaviors, thoughts, coping mechanisms, and ways of expressing themselves change at different stages of their development, deciding what *is* age appropriate is difficult enough in itself. For this reason, deciding when your child's behavior crosses this already-uncertain line is even more of a challenge.

Sometimes, the hardest job a parent has is knowing when *not* to be concerned. As you rear your child from infancy through adolescence, one of your most demanding tasks will be to act quickly and decisively when it's called for and to bite your tongue, hold your breath, and count to ten as many times as necessary to avoid interfering with your child's growth and experience. The hardest part is knowing when to do which.

One factor that makes the process harder is the tendency for parents to pay attention only to the most *annoying* problems. It's natural to do this, but we often place more effort and concern on the merely annoying than we do on the more serious but "quieter" problems.

Throughout this book we'll examine a representative sample of difficulties that your child can experience. As we look at these problems, we'll explore which of them carry immediate dangers or the potential to cause your child serious difficulty in the future. Equally important, you'll learn to differentiate between the signs of immediate danger and those elements of your child's behavior that may well be annoying and even upsetting to you as adults and parents, but that are still relatively normal expressions of childhood.

An example is the tendency of some children toward occasional "crankiness" or being "difficult," contrasted with the child who has oppositional defiant disorder (ODD). Particularly when tired or hungry, many children (and some adults!) will seem cranky and difficult to get along with. Yet the child with ODD, who delights in doing the opposite of whatever you ask him to do and who will argue for any point of view that disagrees with yours (regardless of the consequences to himself), is generally very trying and difficult to be around most of the time.

The tired or hungry child is being just that: a tired or hungry child. The child with ODD, however, can be manifesting serious emotional difficulty that warrants more concern. In this case, a parent would do well to consult with his child's teacher to see how he is doing in school—particularly how he gets along with peers and authority figures. Frank discussions with the parents of a child's friends may also yield valuable information.

In this example, an investigation might reveal that your child is often at odds with his peers, starting arguments and physical fights, being disagreeable and difficult to get along with. His teachers might comment that he has a continual need for direction ("Johnny, stay in your seat and do *not* bother Barbara again!" and "Stop threatening Bill right now!") and that he constantly speaks back to his teacher, defying her attempts to control him.

Or you might find that your child is cranky and difficult just when he's tired, hungry, or doesn't feel well. Children need and deserve to be seen as children, not as shorter, younger versions of adults. Behaviors that are not acceptable for adults are in some cases understandable and reasonable for children, given their relative lack of physical and emotional maturity. Expecting a ten-year-old to be a perfect little gentleman or a perfect little lady is unreasonable and unfair, demanding of your child something that is impossible to deliver.

Our expectations of our children are most frequently based on our own experiences as children. If we were raised by parents who expected us to sit quietly and still in church at five years old, paying rapt attention to the clergyman's words for an hour and a half at a time, there is a good chance we'll expect the same of our children. Of course, you *can* demand that type of behavior from your child, and if your parents expected that of you before you were capable of complying, you might hear yourself saying, "Kids can sit still and behave even at a very young age. After all, I did it, and it didn't ruin me!"

You may be right, of course, to the extent that it didn't ruin you. You coped, like anyone, the best you could. Everyone told your parents what a well-behaved child you were, and you may have come to enjoy the positive attention. Maybe you even learned some other skills. You might, for example, have learned to get strokes (being told you were good, being smiled at) by being a "people pleaser." Even though your normal behavior at that time in your life might really have been more fun-based, less regimented, less disciplined, you learned to squelch your desires early in favor of getting those positive strokes.

Your parents' insistence on your acting grown up before you were ready stole some of your childhood from you, whether you rebelled or went along with the program. Either way, you were prevented from being just a child. If you rebelled, you were often made to feel bad and wrong, even though you were behaving appropriately for a child. If you decided that compliance was the least painful alternative, you were repeatedly reinforced for behavior that denied your true status as a child. Perhaps worse, as a child you couldn't differentiate between things that genuinely pleased you and things that were not really true to your nature but that you did anyway—not to avoid punishment, but to be liked.

As adults, understanding the destructive potential of pushing children to behave at maturity levels they haven't yet achieved is relatively easy to see. All too often parents who were pushed as children, and even parents who weren't pushed as children but who are high achievers and want the same for their children, need to be reminded.   Even though we need to keep our expectations in line with the reality that our children are children, we also need to remember that children rarely progress to higher levels of maturity without the impetus, the push to growth, provided by relationships with peers, teachers, parents, and family.

The Way You View Your Child's Behavior

When looking at your daughter's recent loss of interest in food or the note a teacher sent home about the fight your son started at school, it's important to consider the context of the situation. Here are two different situations for you to consider:

Sally's fourteen-year-old daughter, Julie, had plans to attend her first junior high school dance the next month, but she had been "sidelined" from her active lifestyle for a month because of an injured ankle. She had picked up an extra five or six pounds. Her lack of activity, combined with unchanged eating habits, may have easily resulted in that extra weight.

When Sally noticed that her daughter had little appetite at dinner again one night, she decided to speak privately with Julie after dinner. Concerned about what she might find out, she mentioned that she had noticed that Julie had taken much smaller portions than usual at dinner and that she hadn't had dessert. Sally asked if perhaps she wasn't feeling well.

"Well, Mom, remember how I told you two days ago that my jeans were much tighter than they used to be? Well, I spoke to Mrs. Davis, my health teacher, and asked her if I might have gained some weight because I'd hurt my ankle. She explained that at my age, I have a very active metabolism, and I was very active before I got hurt, so it seemed like I could eat anything I wanted and not gain weight." Sally began to feel somewhat better, but she was still concerned.

Julie continued, saying that Mrs. Davis had explained that lack of physical activity without any change in eating habits probably caused the weight gain. "So, we decided that I'd reduce all my portions just a little bit, and temporarily cut down on desserts, sugar, and fatty foods. Gosh, I hated to pass up your chocolate cake, Mom, it's the best!"

As Julie talked, Sally realized that her daughter was actually very level headed. She had discussed her problem with a knowledgeable adult, and the advice she got would adequately take care of her concerns. Mrs. Davis had apparently been sensitive to Julie's self-image insecurity and handled it appropriately. Mrs. Davis had also taken the time to reinforce Julie's good judgment and had used the situation as an opportunity to explain and reclarify some basic issues of weight control. She had helped Sally's daughter through a challenge—that could have been a problem—by changing it into a learning opportunity.

◇ ◇ ◇

"Johnny, your homeroom teacher, Mr. Gibbon, says in this note that you tried to start a fight with that Williams boy, Blake, and that he had to yell at you to get you to sit down," Sandy said to her son. "What's going on?"

Although he was a fairly good student and hadn't really been a behavioral problem, Sandy had noticed lately that Johnny, or John as he recently seemed to prefer, had been a little irritable. At seventeen, he was a "big kid," tall and muscular, and the girls at school seem to like him . . . which he seemed to like very much.

"Ah, Mom, nothing happened. Uh, I, just got into a little argument with Blake. It was nothing, Mom, honest." Although Mr. Gibbon's note had said that no blows were struck, it still unsettled her to think that he had to yell at Johnny before he would retake his seat.

*She asked him what they had argued about. "Uh, I don't know,"
Johnny started. "It was no big deal . . . I don't even remember what it
was about now." But after seventeen years, Sandy knew when her son
was lying.*

*It took her over half an hour to get Johnny to tell her that he
"really likes Jeannie" and that Blake had been teasing him about his
relationship with her. Worse, Blake liked Jeannie, too, and had asked
her out for Friday night. Although Jeannie had thanked him and said
no, it still angered Johnny that his ex-friend Blake "could do that to
me!" Johnny was obviously angered by the memory and more than a
little embarrassed by his admission, so Sandy decided to talk with
Johnny after he'd completed his homework.*

*Clearly, his thinking, decisions, and actions were not his best, she
thought to herself. On the other hand, this seemed to have been his
first encounter with jealousy over a girl. This wasn't the same type of
jealousy Johnny had felt at Christmas when his brother, Mike, got the
electronic game that Johnny had wanted for months. An opportunity
for an effective discussion of adult-type relationships with her son, ide-
ally involving her husband as well, had presented itself naturally.*

In both scenarios, the attitudes, decisions, and actions of the
children involved could have indicated serious trouble-trouble
that might well have required professional intervention. But by
gently probing to discover the *context* of the observed behavior,
the parents were able to determine the true extent of the problem
and take appropriate action. When that happens, it feels great.
We're proud of ourselves for having the ability to listen, to think
about what has been said, and then to help or find a solution to
the problem. But sometimes, even the best of parents are faced
with situations or troubling emotional or disruptive behavior
that they don't know how to handle. Children's behavior (their
thoughts, ideas, and actions) may completely baffle us—especially if they are out of the realm of what we refer to as normal. We
often attempt to solve the problem or find a way to handle the
misbehavior, but after several attempts over days, even weeks, we
may give up, shake our heads, and walk away. We may talk with
family or friends, ask for their opinions, then try what they suggest. But that doesn't always work, especially if we are trying to
deal with something we don't understand. The inability to
understand our children's behavior creates a dilemma.

When dealing with learning disorders or emotional and

behavioral disorders, unless we are trained or well read in these areas and understand how complex childhood disorders are, we usually don't have the knowledge, skills, or resources needed to treat these problems by ourselves. The resulting feelings of helplessness can become very frustrating and overwhelming. We want to help, but we may not be able to without the intervention of a professional, or several professionals. That may create yet another dilemma for us. To seek outside help, we have to be able to admit first that there is a problem and second, that we don't know how to fix it. To reach out for help then becomes difficult for some parents—involving an outsider in family affairs may seem only to confirm their feelings of helplessness and failure.

It's unfortunate that we enter parenthood with preconceived ideas of what our child will look like, how our child will behave, speak, and even dress. We forget about things like temperament, personality, genetics, environment, and our child's own emerging likes and dislikes, strengths and challenges. We forget about our own temperaments and personalities as parents. We rarely give thought to our own childhood backgrounds and how these factors will influence our child. Our preconceived notions are just that. Rarely is our child just like the child we created in our minds because that image simply lacks all the ingredients. In this book, we are going to take a look at children—these unique individuals capable of giving us so much cause for concern—as well as the many factors that influence their development. This will give you a better idea of why some problems are beyond our ability to mend on our own.

In Julie's and in Johnny's cases there was no need to call a therapist for intervention. With Julie, *no* action might have been a reasonable choice for her mother. Her mother might alternatively have decided to reinforce the good judgment Julie had displayed, but an urgent call to a therapist specializing in teenage eating disorders was not necessary. Teenage girls can become exquisitely sensitive about their weight, and some do go on to develop bulimia. Most do not.

Johnny's situation also offered some hints that major trouble was brewing. Even so, a calm, understanding approach to the problematic behavior revealed that it wasn't so serious that it required a mental health professional to intervene. If we consider his age and maturity level, his response, although ultimately inappropriate, can be understood.

That understanding provides an opening that effective

parents can use to help the child. In this case, it gives Johnny's parents an opportunity to talk with him about caring, romantic relationships with others, the feelings that often go along with those relationships, and more constructive, acceptable, healthy, and helpful ways to deal with them.

Parents who communicate well with their children (by earnestly listening to their concerns, difficulties, hopes, and dreams) and who are active in their children's lives usually have trusting, caring relationships with their children. This type of relationship allows parents to voice their concerns to children and it enables children to feel comfortable sharing with their parents. Actively listening to their child will often tell parents whether they need to be seriously concerned. Probably more often than not, what initially may appear to be a major problem will turn out to be something that concerned and compassionate parents can manage on their own, or with a spouse.

But when the behavior or the mood doesn't change, when the child continues to struggle in school and the parents have tried everything to solve the problem themselves, they are faced with a choice: seek outside help or ignore the situation. It is our hope that this book will enable you to make the right choice, both for your child and for your family.

Which Types of Behaviors May Indicate the Need for Therapy?

Currently in the United States approximately 7.5 million children and adolescents, or twelve percent of all children, suffer from emotional, behavioral, or mental disorders and are in need of professional intervention. Their problems may range from depression to destructive or abusive behaviors to learning disabilities and aggressive acts toward parents or peers. Others may be living in a world of their own—a world of fantasy, magical thinking, or obsessive thoughts. Some problems may be hereditary—they tend to run in families—whereas the cause of other problems may be unknown. Parents should acquaint themselves with the symptoms of the more common emotional, behavioral, psychological, and psychiatric difficulties that are often seen and diagnosed in children. Be suspicious of any of the following behaviors in children. Any one or more of them could indicate the need for therapy.

- A sudden decline in academic performance
- Consistent lying about unimportant things
- Obsessive dwelling on a particular subject
- A sudden and persistent dampening of mood, such as becoming quiet and withdrawn for more than a few days
- A constant display in a preteen or teenager of an "I don't care" attitude
- Exhibition of oppositional behavior at home, in school, or both
- Repetitive behavior that the child seems to have no control over
- Deliberate hurting of others or self
- Displays of total disregard for authority figures
- Displays of hyperactivity, distractibility, and impulsivity
- Comments about not wanting to live or attempts at suicide
- Apparent lack of a sense of right and wrong

- Apparent inability to show empathy or sympathy
- Exhibitions of cruelty toward animals
- Appearance of living in a world of fantasy; exhibitions of magical thinking
- Self-destructive behavior
- Excessive aggression or anger
- Motor or vocal tics
- Severe tamper tantrums
- Stuttering
- Bed-wetting or soiling
- Stealing
- Irritability
- Clinging behaviors
- Persistent fears that are not age appropriate
- Complaints of hearing voices
- Changes in eating or sleep patterns
- Deliberate fire-setting
- Binge eating
- Failure to gain weight due to strict dieting or excessive exercise

Even when your child is clearly displaying one or several of these behaviors, deciding when therapy is needed, which type to pursue, and which class of mental health professionals to consult (psychologist, psychiatrist, social worker, etc.) can be daunting.

Learning about common problems your child might have or develop, as well as how to recognize these problems, what you should do about them, whom you should consult, and which type of therapy is best suited for them are just a few of the issues discussed in this book.

If you suspect that something isn't quite right with your child, this book will equip you with the tools you need to assess and understand your child's behaviors and attitudes more clearly. As parents reading this book, you will be guided to have more understanding than ninety percent of other parents concerning what you must do to ensure your child's academic and emotional well-being. You will learn what can develop within your child, both the good and the not-so-good, and how to reinforce the good you find. School personnel cannot be depended on to perform this important task alone. Every child is only one of many at school, although teachers are often the first to notice that a child is experiencing some sort of difficulty. Ultimately, parents must be responsible for learning about normal childhood development and for recognizing when something appears not so right with their children.

TWO

The Many Roots of Childhood Problems

Watching a child struggle can be frustrating, painful, and heart wrenching for parents. Even worse is not understanding why. Why is she so fearful? Why is he always brooding in his room instead of playing outside with the other children? Why does he always blink his eyes or twitch like he does? Why can't he sit still? Why does she hide behind me when a friend or a stranger approaches? Why can't he look anyone in the eye when he's spoken to? Why won't she eat? Why the tantrums or aggressive behavior? Why does he not understand humor, jokes, puns? Why did he blow up at his teacher today? Why, indeed!

Who's to Blame?

With each question, we wonder and we worry. Sometimes we even laugh as we remember the words of a parent, usually our mother: "Someday you will have children of your own and then you'll understand." So here we are, all grown up with children of our own, only we don't understand. Well, some things we really do understand, like loving our children more than ourselves, but when something appears not quite right with our children, we often look at the problem and wonder if we've done or said something to cause this unusual fear, this dreadful behavior, this physical aggression. After all, we all know that parents are to blame for most of the problems that children experience, right? Wrong! Unfortunately, however, most people, including many parents and even some mental health professionals, still believe this. In fact, according to a survey conducted by the National Institute of Mental Health in 1990, sixty-five percent of the people who responded believe that bad parenting causes mental illness!

How much easier it is to accept a physical disability that we can understand without judging the parents, like the child born with cerebral palsy, Down syndrome, or a heart condition. But even in cases like these, fingers are occasionally pointed and words whispered: "The poor child. Wonder what his mother did during her pregnancy?" Admittedly, substance abuse, smoking, and lack of prenatal care can cause birth defects, but not all mothers are guilty of harming the fetus. Sometimes, for whatever reason, the child is born with a disability. It is no one's fault. Other times the disability is hidden but biologically based, as in the case of a learning disorder or an emotional disorder. Again, no one is to blame—not Mom, not Dad, and certainly not the child.

But what happens to us when we watch a ten-year-old child acting out in public, openly and loudly defying his parents? Some of us may shudder. We might even swear that we'll never have a child like that. We're amazed that the child's parents let her get away with this behavior. Why don't they discipline her, we wonder. And what about the eight-year-old who throws himself onto the floor, crying and screaming in a full-blown temper tantrum? What a spoiled brat, we think. That's his parents' fault for giving in to him all the time. What he needs is a good spanking and someone to show him who's the boss. And what about a fifteen-year-old who shouts obscenities as he's walking through the mall? How many of us immediately question what his parents must be like? "Can you imagine the language that must be used in his home?" we might comment.

With physical disabilities—disabilities that we can see—the blame is rarely placed on the parents. Emotional and behavioral problems found in children deserve the same respect. In the first situation mentioned, the acting-out child has been diagnosed with both oppositional defiant disorder and a learning disorder (LD). The eight-year-old, who has lost control of himself and is in the midst of a temper tantrum, has a low tolerance level. He's impulsive and hyperactive, frequently demands attention, and is easily frustrated. It's not always easy for him to accept "no" for an answer. He also needs high degrees of stimulation, more than most children, and when that is not available, he often creates his own—all signs and symptoms of attention deficit hyperactivity disorder (ADHD). The third child, who screams out obscenities, could have a rare, complex vocal tic called coprolalia, found in less than ten percent of individuals with Tourette's disorder. (These disorders will be discussed in more detail later in this book.) Are the parents to be blamed for something they could not control?

Although parents can exacerbate the symptoms of oppositional defiant disorder by ineffective discipline, they cannot "cause" it to occur; far too many other factors are involved—factors that will be discussed throughout the book. ADHD is almost always inherited; the behaviors are not learned. Parents can increase or decrease the severity of some of the symptoms, but again, they are not to blame. The same holds true for Tourette's disorder. It is no one's fault! We emphasize this because too many parents blame themselves for things they have absolutely no power or control over, which can distract them from dealing with their child's problem constructively and effectively.

Childhood Disorders

Only recently have parents and the general public begun to learn that disorders such as depression, phobias, attention deficit hyperactivity disorder, and anxiety disorders are medical problems found in children. Previously, only physicians and scientists were aware of these problems in children. The medical information that once was available only to medical professionals is now easily available to us—and written so that the layperson can understand it. That's the good news. However, most parents don't read the information that is available, so when problems with our children develop—and all children have some problems, if only minor—we're at a loss. We know something isn't right, but we have no idea what's wrong or what to do about it.

Many of us will pick up a book on childhood illnesses or read some articles on ear infections or toilet training, but how many of us actually seek information on emotional, behavioral, or learning disorders in children? How many parents know the signs and symptoms of childhood depression? Apparently, not enough of us. Studies of children between the ages of six and twelve have shown that as many as one child in ten suffers from depression—and unfortunately, most go untreated. A survey by the Institute of Medicine of the National Academy of Sciences estimates that seventeen to twenty-two percent of all children have emotional problems such as anxiety disorders, mood disorders, ADHD, and psychoses.

Some parents may not give much thought to childhood emotional or behavioral disorders until they begin to suspect that their child is a bit different from other children, or school problems develop, or a friend or relative points out that maybe "something isn't quite right." Even then some parents are reluctant to draw attention to the problem. Many parents wonder what they did wrong. They may worry that they are to blame, and they don't want to encounter their own fear. Or they may worry that their child will be labeled as mentally ill or sick if he receives treatment.

Or perhaps many of us do think of the possibility but prefer to think that it can't happen to our child. We know children will have colds, flu, and ear infections; we accept that effortlessly. Unconsciously we also know that no one will blame *us* for our child's cold or flu because these are common illnesses in children. It is much harder for us to accept that our children may also be vulnerable to illnesses and disorders that we feel may stigmatize them—or for which we might be blamed.

What We Are Learning

Concern about children's health has been on the increase, but we are still a long way from understanding children's mental health. Of the twelve million children suffering from mental illness, fewer than one in five receives treatment. Yet, in comparison, seventy-four percent of children with physical disabilities receive treatment.

For years it was thought that children did not suffer from emotional or mental problems because childhood was a happy, carefree time of life. Children, it was believed, did not have stresses like those of adults. We have since learned that this is not true. According to the American Psychiatric Association,"between 200,000 and 300,000 children suffer from autism, a pervasive developmental disorder that appears in the first three years of life. Millions suffer from learning disorders, attention deficit disorder, attachment disorders, conduct disorders, and substance abuse."

The results of two surveys mentioned in the December 1988 issue of *Archives of General Psychiatry* indicated that a large percentage of children—approximately one in five—have moderate to severe psychiatric disorders. In one study of a group of 789 children, ages seven to eleven, who presented high scores for emotional and behavioral problems, twenty-two percent had one psychiatric disorder or more. Of these, phobias, oppositional defiant disorder, overanxious disorder, and separation anxiety disorder were the most frequent diagnoses.

Researchers have little idea what happens to children with psychiatric disorders who go untreated as they reach adulthood, but we do know that therapy, medications, parental knowledge and guidance, and so on can assist children to lead a better life now and in the future. Early intervention is extremely significant, and it may also stave off higher costs (monetary and otherwise) to both individuals and society down the road.

Genetics and Other Biological Factors

Not so long ago, most emotional and behavioral problems of children were blamed on faulty parenting styles and the relationship between parent and child. Thus, if a child had behavioral or emotional problems, the parents were seen as negligent, remiss, or even abusive. Pity the competent parent who had a "bad kid"! Now we understand that although family environment will contribute to a child's problems, the home environment is only one aspect of a multidimensional picture. Mental health professionals speak of behavioral and emotional problems as being "multifactorial in their determinants," which simply means that those problems have two or more causes. One cause is rarely sufficient to bring on the problem or disorder—the causes are complex, and many include a biological component that places the child at risk. This doesn't mean that if your uncle wet the bed until he was seventeen that your son will do the same. Nor does it mean that if Aunt Jenny has bipolar disorder that one of your children will eventually be diagnosed with bipolar disorder. It means only that your child is at a higher risk than the little boy down the street who has no history of bipolar disorder or bed-wetting on either side of his family. A child whose parent has been diagnosed as having an antisocial personality disorder is at greater risk of being antisocial himself. This is not inevitable, however, because there are multiple factors involved, such as the child's temperament, peer group, family relationships, and the family's economic status, to name just a few.

We now have a better understanding of genetics and the importance of heredity—the genetic transmission of characteristics from parent to child. We know that some disorders are transmitted from parent to child, and we know that one grandparent may have had the same or similar problem—or maybe it was Uncle Harry, who everyone loved, but who couldn't ever sit down long enough to relax. Sometimes a parent can look at her child and say, "He's just like my mother, always anxious about something." When a child is having problems, and we recognize that someone else in our family has or had the same problem, it makes the diagnosis easier to establish—we are able to provide a physician with reliable family background information—even if Uncle Harry was never diagnosed for his hyperactivity. The drawback, however, is that if Uncle Harry's behavior appeared completely "normal" because several other family members displayed the same traits, a parent may not recognize that those traits may represent a medical disorder.

Although we've just discussed the multifactorial nature of serious disorders, and we know that many of those factors are not genetic/biological, let's focus more closely for a moment on these biological components. To gain a better understanding of the biological component and how varied its effects on the child can be, we'll look first at genetics, one type of biological influence, as if it were the only determinant. Then we'll consider some of the other biological components as if they were the only important factors.

Genetics

When we speak of genetics, most people think "either you have the gene for it, or you don't," whichever trait, good or bad, is under discussion. In reality, it's almost never that simple.

An easy way to understand this is to think of the genetic code of our DNA as blueprints for building first the parts of a complex, modern automobile and then for building the automobile itself. Anyone who's ever owned a car that was a lemon (or has had to listen to someone who did!) can realize that even with perfect plans, there are a lot of steps between the plan and the final product.

Even with "good" genes then, things can happen. "Glitches" can occur, and a child might have a problem that he wasn't genetically destined for. Similarly, a child born with genes that should have resulted in a specific disorder may never develop it.

To be more biologically accurate then, we speak of a "genetic predisposition" toward developing a certain disorder. Just having the genes for a specific disorder does not mean the child will develop it. And if the child does develop it, it might not express itself fully—the child could experience the problem more mildly than is usually seen. So, a child may be genetically predisposed toward an emotional, developmental, or behavior disorder, but he may or may not develop it. Or he may develop it to a greater or lesser degree than other members of his family.

Before we leave the discussion of genetics and move on to other biological factors, we need to examine the situation in which a child is born with the genetic blueprint to predispose him toward a specific disorder. The blueprint is faithfully followed, there are no glitches, yet he never develops the disorder. How can this be?

Earlier, we said that there can be mistakes in the execution of the plan; the blueprint is perfectly followed, but somehow, the biological mechanism charged with following the blueprint doesn't work perfectly. When that happens, the good genes (good parts of the plan) may not be expressed properly, having a serious negative effect or possibly having no noticeable effect at all.

Similarly, a bad gene (a part of the plan that, if followed, should result in a serious problem) also may not have the expected impact on the "final product." Even though we would anticipate that gene to cause a serious problem, it might not have any noticeable effect, or its negative effect may be comparatively minor. But in this case, we know the child has the bad gene; we also know that there were no mistakes in the body's factories. They followed the plan exactly, and everything worked perfectly. Even so, he developed normally, without the problem. Why? To solve this mystery, we need to go back to the multifactorial nature of the disorders we're discussing, limiting it, for now, to just genetics.

It turns out that not only do many factors come together to cause these disorders, but also many of these factors, including genetic ones, are themselves multifactorial. In this case, the child had a genetic predisposition to the problem that needed to be activated by something else, but that "something else" never came along!

How this works is illustrated well by that serious disease, alcoholism. It has been well established that certain people inherit a gene that greatly increases the likelihood that they will develop alcoholism; yet some of those people never become alcoholics. The reason is actually quite simple. They just don't drink!

They may, for example, belong to a religion that frowns on consuming alcohol, and so they don't. Or they may have other moral conditioning against alcohol. They may have thought about their family history, considered that a large number of their relatives were alcoholics, and decided not to take a chance—they never started drinking. Even though they may have grown up with all the other factors (social, psychological, economic, etc.), and had actually inherited the genes that placed them at even higher risk, they still didn't develop the problem.

Even genetic inheritance isn't infallible. Contrary to what many people think, even a child's having the genetic predisposition to certain disorders doesn't always mean that we cannot help to change his destiny to one far better.

Listing and discussing all the other biological factors that can influence the development of serious emotional and behavioral disorders in children would be enormous tasks in themselves and are beyond the scope and purpose of this book. Even if we disregard for the moment the long-term, negative emotional effects that some youngsters growing up with a physical disability eventually display (and not all children with disabilities or challenges do; none *need* to), there are still some biological factors that merit mentioning.

Mother's Health During Pregnancy

At this point in the history of humankind it shouldn't be necessary even to mention how important a mother's health is to her unborn child; regrettably, it still is. During the first trimester, much of the important work of organogenesis is completed; this is the beginning work on the construction of all the internal organs, including the brain. An incredibly complex, sensitive mass of tissue, the brain is the "hardware" of our body's "computer"; our experiences, training, and environment constitute the "software." A computer with faulty wiring and bad connections doesn't work as it was intended, regardless of how wonderful or perfect is the software it's loaded with. If a mother is in ill health during her pregnancy, eating poorly, and consuming alcohol or other drugs, her child's computer, his brain, will not work as it was intended.

Nutrition

After the child is born, his nutrition remains very important. In poverty-stricken regions of the world, many children suffer life-long, devastating intellectual and emotional consequences from lack of food. Both types of inadequate diets—those that are too low in total calories, as well as those that contain too little protein for children's metabolic and anabolic (tissue-building) needs—condemn children to adult lives of intellectual inadequacy and emotional impoverishment. In fact, maternal health and nutrition during pregnancy and the nutrition of young children are two of the most significant factors determining a person's future as a child and an adult.

Early Emotional and Sensory Stimulation

First demonstrated convincingly many years ago, it's an accepted truth in the medical and scientific communities that early physical stimulation—that is, being held and touched—can be crucial to normal development, both physiologically and emotionally. Being held, fed, bathed, groomed, and even played with all stimulate the growth of the young human brain. Stimulation also activates the associative and networking capacities of that organ. Studies on children who were raised in orphanages in war-torn parts of Europe during and after World War II and studies on other children raised at the same time but in different, more normal circumstances were very revealing. If one reviews those studies—acknowledging that corrections for differences in diet and many other factors will always be less than perfect—the data are most convincing. The emotionally warm touch of a loving adult, with much smiling and playing, stimulation and activity, was crucial to normal emotional and intellectual development. Not surprisingly, studies conducted in the United States fifty years later confirm these findings in institutionalized children born in foreign countries—toddlers, preschoolers, and school-age children who later were placed for adoption with families in the United States.

Of course, there are many, many other biological factors, as we mentioned earlier. And it remains important to remember some other key factors. For example, an otherwise physiologically healthy child might have diabetes, kidney problems, heart or liver ailments, or other serious illness, none of which necessarily causes intellectual or emotional problems. Even so, these important biological factors may well have serious consequences for the child, indirectly causing intellectual problems such as learning disabilities or other problems with cognition. Emotional and behavioral problems may develop, either as a direct result of the illness's effects on the brain or, indirectly, as a result of the depression that can stem from a serious or life-threatening disease. Poor self-image and low self-esteem can result from serious illness, as they can from physical disability.

Here are some important conclusions:

- As important as genetics can be in predisposing our children toward certain outcomes, good or bad, there are myriad other biological factors, many of which are as important as genetic inheritance.

- Biological factors are, in general, complex and variable.

- Genetic inheritance in particular, although it can predispose, is beyond any individual's ability to control.

- Awareness of biological factors, especially genetic inheritance, can work powerfully to relieve inappropriate parental guilt.

- Equally important, if your child has biological factors that negatively influence his emotional health or behavior, your knowledge of those factors and your appropriate intervention can improve the quality of your child's life today and help assure for him the brightest future. With the help of qualified mental health professionals and medical assistance as needed, your understanding of his problems may be the most important asset he has in receiving the care he needs.

Compare an emotional or behavioral disorder to a physical disorder: A child who has lost three grandparents and an aunt to cancer is at greater risk for developing cancer than a child with no family history of cancer. Unfortunately, we seem to be more understanding, sympathetic, and approving of the parent who has a child with cancer than of the parent who has a child with an emotional or behavioral disorder or a mental illness—even if we're that parent!

Temperament and Goodness of Fit

We must also take into account the temperament of the child. By *temperament* we mean the child's inborn response pattern or style (those mental and emotional qualities that distinguish individuals from one another). Some children are just naturally shy; some are good humored; others are outgoing; still others are extremely energetic and taxing.

Some theorists believe that behavior problems can arise when a child's temperament is opposite that of his parents. For instance, when parents are quiet types, good natured and easygoing, and have a child who is energetic, defiant, and impulsive, behavior problems can develop. Theorists would then question the "goodness of fit" between parent and child. Some laid-back parents may actually enjoy and appreciate having a rambunctious child—the child brightens the somewhat solemn mood of the home. Thus, the fit between parent and child is recognized as "good."

But another parent may not cope well with this type of child. Instead of accepting the child as he is, the parent tries to squelch the child's natural response (his temperament), hoping to make the child more like her. This may be done consciously or unconsciously, but no matter; there is then a "poor fit" between parent and child. Without intervention, the result of this "poor fit" can have damaging effects on the child because he cannot meet the expectations of his parent. The child may then either rebel and act out or become withdrawn and depressed.

Still other parents may feel they are somehow to blame for the child's temperament. The resulting guilt leads them to parent inconsistently, even hesitantly. Again, there is a "poor fit" between the child's temperament and the parents' temperament. Behavioral and emotional problems often develop as a result.

New behaviors can be learned, however, and incorporated into the child's temperament. A child who is shy by temperament, for instance, may learn to benefit from not being so shy. For example, if she learns to make new and interesting friends and to have positive experiences formerly prevented by her shyness, she may, over time, change in temperament to become someone who is more outgoing.

Environment

Indisputably, environment also plays a substantial role in the development of some types of emotional and behavioral problems. Children who come from families who are in constant conflict, or in which the children are not held accountable for their actions, or where parents are overly protective or too lenient, undeniably are influenced by such environments. An overprotective parent is afraid that his child will fail and not be able to get back up on his own, so he shields the child from the realities of life, and thus the child is unable to learn from his mistakes, to make decisions, or to form his own identity. Lenient parents often want to be more like friends than parents, so setting limits is difficult—they fear losing the child's love, or they may believe that children should have freedom to grow without boundaries. Children need and want firm limits (applied fairly), consistency, structure, and routine. They also need love and affection. In fact, they need all these things to grow into healthy individuals, just as they need different limits on their behavior as they move from one stage of development to the next.

Often it's difficult to differentiate between which behavior problems are caused by inadequate parenting skills (for instance, the parents' response or lack of response to the child) and which behavior problems are caused by the effect the child has on the parents (the response the child evokes from the parents). Parents of anxious children, for instance, are often overly protective. The question then becomes this: Is the child anxious because the parents are overly protective, or is the child's anxiety the reason the parents feel the need to protect and keep the child from harm?

The home environment should be a safe refuge for family members, but instead it may be filled with substance-abuse problems, financial difficulties, communication and problem-solving deficits, marital conflict, divorce, isolation, alienation, unemployment or job-related pressures, or psychiatric problems. As well, the school environment should be safe, but in many schools in the United States it is not. Gangs of hoodlums walk the halls with weapons, defying teachers, and bullying students. Children become anxious, afraid to go to school. Children may have undiagnosed learning disabilities or attention deficit hyperactivity disorder (ADHD), making school a dreaded place to go each day and resulting in acting-out behaviors in the home or in the classroom. Any of these situations in the home or school environment can exacerbate or even cause psychiatric disorders such as anxiety disorders, phobias, or mood disorders.

Not to be forgotten are children's peers. Peers can be an extraordinary gift to our children, or they can be a natural disaster waiting to happen. Children with learning problems or with emotional or behavioral disorders often have low self-esteem, particularly those children who are undiagnosed and untreated. As a result they may lack adequate social skills, which hinders them from making or keeping friends. They may act much younger for their age than do their peers, or they may be labeled as "dumb" or "stupid" by their classmates. Children with low self-esteem who appear "different" to their peers often end up running with the wrong group of friends because it is the only group that doesn't exclude them.

Our point again is that many factors contribute to the development of emotional and behavioral disorders. As parents we must keep this in mind. Too often, we want to blame ourselves; we feel guilty. Whether or not a parent realizes that the guilt is inappropriate doesn't matter. Most of us can't help asking ourselves, "Did I do something to cause this?" Or we try to think of a situation that might have triggered the problem: "Maybe I started toilet training too soon, or maybe it was the day when I got so angry with Eric for breaking the window." The guilt can become a real problem for parents who can't seem to stop blaming themselves. We must remember that our children develop in a world in which many factors affect them. We are not the sole influences on their lives. Although it's natural for parents to go through the stages of grief—one of which is blaming themselves—when their child is diagnosed with any type of medical problem, the key is to not get stuck too long in any one stage, but rather to move forward to acceptance. After parents are able to accept the diagnosis, they can move into an advocacy position and work for the child.

Maybe All Is Not As It Seems

Not every problem that erupts in childhood is labeled a "disorder." Some problems, like depression, are often temporary and directly related to special circumstances, such as divorce, a move to a new home, or the birth of a sibling. A child whose parents are going through a divorce may struggle in school for a year or two, her grades may drop, and her parents and teachers may be worried. Does she have a learning disorder that is suddenly surfacing? Chances are good that she doesn't. She may, however, be overstressed, worried, anxious, or depressed and, as a result, be unable to concentrate on schoolwork. After the situation is resolved and her life settles down, she is usually able to bounce back and be the good student she was before. Oftentimes a problem may be behavior typical of the child's age. It may even be worse than in most children of the same age, but still be within the normal range. And frequently, as quickly as the problem seemed to erupt, it ends. The child has progressed to another stage of development.

Sometimes, however, children with even temporary emotional or behavioral difficulties need professional intervention. As parents we may know what is causing the behavior (for example, he's jealous of the new baby), but we're too close to the problem to see the solution. Or we've attempted several approaches, but nothing we've tried has worked. A parent may need to meet with a therapist for only one or two sessions to find a solution. If the child continues to have difficulties or if his mood hasn't changed, the therapist will probably want to see the child as well. Problems that develop because of unusual circumstances are addressed in chapter seven.

Looking Ahead

Although it would be impossible for us to identify in this book every problem that could develop with your child, in the next few chapters we have examined some of the most common problems and childhood disorders and presented the signs and symptoms with which parents should be familiar. We've given you current criteria, and we hope that the information provided can help you identify what's going on with your child.

If you don't see your child in chapters three or four, but your gut feeling is that something is truly wrong, we urge you to seek help from a mental health professional immediately. If your child has been diagnosed with a disorder, but you're not satisfied that the diagnosis is correct, or if you feel that something else is going on with your child in addition to what has been diagnosed, we urge you to go with your intuition and continue to seek help. Obtain a second or even a third opinion. If, however, there is a consensus from two or three therapists, question your reasons for not believing the diagnosis. You may be in denial about a situation that will not improve until it is faced.

It is our hope that this book will help parents who are distraught about their children, parents who may have already asked their parents, grandparents, friends, and others for advice, believing that they are doing something wrong and that the advice they've been given just hasn't helped. If you are a parent who has been told by your mother, baby-sitter, a teacher, or even a neighbor that your child is acting strangely, or if deep down inside you have concerns that you haven't voiced to anyone, we hope you will find the guidance you need in these pages to make the right decisions about your child and his future.

THREE

Does Your Child Need Therapy?

E ven competent, educated, and tuned-in parents may not recognize that their child has a behavioral, emotional, or learning problem. Knowing common warning signs, as mentioned in
chapter one, can assist in determining if your child could benefit
from the intervention of a mental health professional. Not all
behavioral or emotional problems are serious disorders, or even
disorders at all. Often they are temporary problems, the result of
special circumstances (see chapter seven). But sometimes the
problem is, unfortunately, a real medical problem. The good
news is that the earlier the child is diagnosed and treated, the
better the outcome.

You may be thinking, "What if I'm not sure? What if this
is just a phase she's going through?" Recognizing that a child is
in trouble is not always easy. Parents have to understand what is
normal for their child's age—for example, temper tantrums are
normal for a two-year-old—and for their child's disposition. But
when an eight-year-old is having temper tantrums every time he
doesn't get his own way, that's not matter-of-course unless there
are unusual circumstances presently in his life and he's reacting
to those events. If the child has never stopped having temper
tantrums, and if the tantrums are actually worse in intensity and
duration than when he was younger, the child is in trouble.

Anytime a behavior is displayed too frequently, too severely,
or at the wrong time or place, it's a signal that help is needed. If
you're still not sure if your concern is justified, talk with parents
of children the same age as your child, your child's teacher, or
your child's pediatrician. Be cautious if you are told that "this is
just a phase" or that "he'll grow out of it," especially if you've
been concerned for a while. Some problems and some disorders
don't just fade away—common problems, like ADHD or learning

disorders, last a lifetime. Children with such problems will have tremendous difficulties keeping up in school and relating socially to peers without professional intervention and treatment. Other problems, such as depression, anxiety, and phobias, can be treated, often resulting in a lessening or removal of symptoms.

A child who is having difficulties, usually behavioral, in more than one area (camp, home, school, in the neighborhood, in after-school care, or during extracurricular activities)—you know because your phone is always ringing as you are told of the latest episodes involving your child—is in trouble. Difficulties may include such things as aggressive behavior toward peers, inability to keep his hands to himself, impulsive behavior requiring constant supervision, intentionally harming others, or smashing or stealing property belonging to friends and classmates.

A child whose emotional responses suddenly change (for instance, a child who worries excessively about school or other concerns that she didn't worry about before, or who is short, irritable, defiant, or oppositional) is distressed and not coping well. Similarly, a child who experiences functional changes, such as making failing grades, not maintaining friendships, neglecting grooming and self-care, and showing no interest in pursuing hobbies or sports normally enjoyed is sending out a plea for help. When a shy twelve-year-old whose teacher asks her a question abruptly shouts, "Damn it, leave me alone" and stomps out of the classroom, she, too, is making an appeal for assistance and support. Something just isn't right. The "symptom" is a plea for help. The child's symptom, in the case of the twelve-year-old, has crossed the line of what is defined as normal behavior in school.

If you witness persistent problems (grades have continued to decline, he's becoming more and more aggressive, she has no friends), if the problems are causing disruptions in more than one place, if you notice emotional or functional changes, or if the behavior of the child is disturbing to you, then go with your gut feeling. Your intuition is telling you something is wrong. Your concerns are, no doubt, warranted.

Mothers today still spend more time on average with their children than fathers do, providing care and attending to their daily needs, so they are particularly good observers of the emotional, social, and behavioral aspects of their children. They may not know what the specific problem is, but they know when something is out of sync.

It's essential to remember that a child with any type of disorder is extremely dependent on you to recognize warning signs and to seek professional intervention. Without your recognition and help, your child can easily fall through the cracks both academically and socially. An undiagnosed and untreated childhood disorder interferes with the child's normal development, attacks the child's self-esteem, and unfortunately, can set the stage for a lifetime of struggle. No one ever said that parenting is easy! It can be downright frightening at times, especially when we're observing distressing behaviors in a child whom we love immensely.

Some Common Warning Signs at Specific Ages

Although you certainly don't want to run immediately to the doctor with every troublesome behavior you observe, warning signs such as those we discussed earlier serve as red flags. Not all situations are as clear cut as we would hope because at each stage of development children face a variety of challenges. However, knowing which behaviors are age appropriate (in comparison with other children the same age) and which are not can help you decide if your child really does need help.

Preschool Years
Seek help if your youngster is having problems with any of the following: difficulty playing with friends because of unacceptable behaviors such as aggression; no children want to play with him; impulsive or hyperactive behavior; does not have normal fears (not afraid of climbing a bookcase, jumping into a swimming pool without knowing how to swim); has extremely long temper tantrums; shows no interest in learning, even if it's just how to count to five; has speech or language difficulties; has abnormal fears; is always bored; can't be left alone for even a few moments; is extremely demanding, overly anxious, hot tempered, abnormally fearful of people or situations, or displays signs of any of the disorders outlined in chapters four or five. Keep in mind that in the preschool years, most children will display many of these types of behavior just because they *are* children. It is only when the behavior is too intense, too frequent, that it becomes a problem for the child.

If you feel frustrated, feel depressed much of the time because of your child's behavior, and begin to question if you are capable of parenting your child, you should seek assistance. There could be a number of reasons you are having difficulty parenting, including depression, unachieved expectations of parenthood or of your child, caring for a difficult child, and so forth. Young children rarely need to be in therapy. However, for parents, a few sessions with a psychologist, psychiatrist, or other mental health worker specializing in helping parents develop positive parenting techniques and coping skills can be helpful. Sometimes a change in parenting style can greatly reduce difficulties with a child. If behaviors persist, the therapist may want to see your child. Either way you have a valuable resource to call upon if problems persist.

School-Age Children
Signs that may indicate a problem in school-age children include the following: she has difficulty learning (she appears to be "lazy," "slow," or unmotivated, complains that the schoolwork is too hard); despite an average or above-average IQ she is significantly behind in some subjects but at grade level or higher in others; she can make friends but is unable to keep them; she doesn't want to go to school or refuses to go; she is consistently irritable, anxious, moody, defiant, uncooperative, angry, or aggressive toward friends, adults, parents, and teachers; she is extremely shy; she prefers being alone; she won't take "no" for an answer; she appears to have obsessive thoughts or compulsive actions; she doesn't understand humor, jokes, or puns; she has self-care skills that are behind age level; she has difficulty sleeping; she has persistent trouble with nightmares, bedwetting, stealing, fire-setting; or she exhibits signs of any disorders outlined in chapters four or five.

Preteens
Beginning in the preadolescent years, fitting in and being accepted are very important. Seek help if your child admits that he has no friends—he's concerned and searching for reasons why. Short-term therapy to learn more appropriate social skills may be necessary. If he displays any of the behaviors listed for school-age children—including but not limited to distorted thinking, unusual behaviors, eating problems, or school absenteeism—always consult with a mental health professional. Remember that teachers are also a valuable source of information in any age group and can provide important insight about the child in the school set-

ting. If you don't hear from a teacher, don't assume that no problem behaviors are being displayed in school. Always ask.

Teenagers

The teen years can be difficult for both parents and children. Because teenagers are seeking to establish their identity and decrease their dependence on their parents, peers usually become their confidants. Although your daughter may have always come to you with her concerns, she now looks to her peers for advice, making it sometimes difficult for you to know if she is experiencing any specific problems in her social life or in school. Seek outside help if your child refuses to talk with you, or if you notice depression (or any drastic change in mood), an abnormal amount of noncompliance (failure to follow school or house rules), changes in sleeping patterns, or absenteeism from school. Also seek help if you suspect the use of drugs, notice unusual weight gain or loss, or if the teen has difficulties in several areas of life (school, home, social activities, camp, etc.), or any of the symptoms discussed in chapters four or five.

Dealing with the Emotions

Most parents do their best to meet the needs of their children. They ensure that their children are fed, clothed, and educated, and when their children are ill, parents try to find the best in medical attention. Most parents, however, feel inadequate when it comes to recognizing and dealing effectively with emotional or psychological difficulties because they often lack training in this area. The task of learning about all the problems children might have or might develop is overwhelming, and most parents simply do not have the time to read volumes of literature on childhood disorders.

Despite the best intentions to meet all the needs of their children, when emotional, academic, or behavioral problems develop that parents aren't prepared to handle, few parents immediately think of seeking professional psychological or psychiatric care. There are many reasons for this.

Fear

Fear is perhaps one of the most important reasons parents give little thought to seeking psychological or psychiatric assistance. Parents may never have had any experience with mental and emotional problems before. Their apprehension, coupled with a lack of experience and knowledge, may prevent them from acknowledging that their child has difficulties. In such cases, parents fear that their child is "crazy" or at least that the child is somehow "defective." This trepidation may forestall parents from discussing the problems with the child's pediatrician, preventing the child from receiving the immediate professional help he may desperately need. "No passion so effectually robs the mind of all its powers of acting and reasoning as fear," said Edmund Burke, a British philosopher of the eighteenth century. Fear alone can prevent even the most intelligent parent from seeking professional intervention.

Having emotional or psychological difficulties as a child need not be a predictor of future problems. In fact, regardless of the type or severity of the difficulties your child may be experiencing, early and effective treatment is the single best way you can prevent future problems. Some parents, unable to accept that their "perfect" child has difficulties requiring professional help, make matters far worse by denying that reality.

Concern about Labeling

Many parents worry that if they seek professional help for their child's psychological problems, the child may be labeled by school officials and others as "troubled," "difficult," "disturbed," or even "sick." Although that has been a realistic fear in years past, parents can now insist on more sensitive treatment of their child's problems, including the protection of confidentiality.

Although most parents would rather not have their child labeled as having a "disorder"—obsessive-compulsive disorder, attention deficit hyperactivity disorder, oppositional defiant disorder, or depression, for instance—it is far better to have a label that explains the "whys" of peculiar behaviors than to have the child labeled as stupid, crazy, difficult, or weird, especially within the academic setting. A diagnosis permits a child to receive educational services and treatment strategies that he may greatly benefit from but that are not accessible without a diagnosis.

Lack of Knowledge

Regrettably, with all the time and effort put into education by public service advertising aimed at educating parents about the medical problems and needs of their children, comparatively little exposure and educational effort are expended to help parents understand mental illness in children. The generally negative connotation of the term *mental illness* also prevents many from dealing head-on with these types of difficulties.

As a result, it is hardly surprising that many parents are woefully unprepared to deal effectively with their children when they notice that "something isn't quite right." Where there is a lack of knowledge, denial, the process by which we persistently refuse to acknowledge a serious problem even in the face of incontrovertible evidence, can take over and protect many parents from having to deal with the reality of their children's problems.

Denial

Denial is a defense mechanism that all of us have experienced at one time or another. Often, it is the initial response to hearing bad news that is overwhelming. Although staying in denial would be unhealthy and prolong our suffering upon hearing of, say, a parent's death, it is a natural first response to the unthinkable. It often serves to give us an opportunity to gird ourselves for the true impact of extremely troubling realities.

Most often the parent who denies a child's problem inappropriately sees the problem as an expression of the parent's personal failure. "If my child has a problem, I must be a bad parent. I don't want to feel that I'm a bad parent, so my child can't have a problem." The problem that the child is having may or may not have to do with the parenting skills of Mom or Dad.

A more mature response to learning that a child has problems is for the parent to first acknowledge that reality. Even if a parent can think of situations or times when he may have inadvertently contributed to that problem, the primary emphasis needs to be placed on present realities: the *child's* needs. That is, a problem exists—now. It needs to be dealt with before it gets worse, causes other problems, or sets the child up for a difficult future.

"But what if I feel guilty?"

Guilt is an emotion that, by itself, accomplishes little except punishment. However, it can serve as an impetus to change, and when it does, it serves its purpose best when it is brief, leading directly to effective action.

New parenting skills can be learned, and old parenting skills can be modified to be more effective. You hurt yourself as well as your child by denying your child's problem because it threatens your self-esteem. If you or your spouse tends to deny your child's problem when it "comes too close to home," keep in mind that you may be unintentionally preventing your child from receiving the help he needs while you are protecting your own feelings.

If you recognize that you tend to deny your children's problems, acknowledge this to your child's helping professional as a possible complicating factor when presenting your child's situation. It will help the professional be more effective with your child. Then, as the professional counsels you on how best to support your child, she will also be able to assist you with your feelings.

If you have denied your child's problems in the past, although it may not have been the most positive thing you've ever done, it is a very human and understandable thing to do. But feeling guilty just compounds the error. Instead, be glad you've realized a more advantageous way to deal with his needs, helping him rather than making the problem worse. Helping your child is sometimes the best way to help yourself.

Doubting Parenting Abilities

Not only are most parents unprepared to handle their children's emotional, academic, or behavioral problems, but also the first thought that usually enters their mind is that in some way they are responsible for the problems the child is encountering. Did they not give enough quality time through the years? Did they push the child too hard to succeed above and beyond others of the same age? Or did that two-week vacation they took when their daughter was only two leave lasting scars? In other words, they question their parenting abilities. After all, some parents ask, how could such vexatious behaviors surface if they were doing their job properly?

Unfortunately, friends and relatives may also be suspicious of parents whose children exhibit unusual problems, causing even more parental guilt. Rather than support loved ones, some extended family members and even close friends, frightened by what they observe, may turn away just when parents need their assistance most.

Acceptance Is Difficult

It's difficult to accept that your child may have a problem, especially if he was born healthy. You don't expect that your child will have problems that will interfere with his development. So when you begin to suspect that he is extremely depressed or anxious, or has a behavioral disorder, denial reaches in and grabs you. This denial relieves you for a while. Then reality strikes again when a teacher, relative, or a friend makes a comment about your child. Parents of children with any type of disorder will mention that denial, but they are always quick to add that they "always knew something was wrong, or different" long before someone else told them.

Fathers seem to have more difficulty accepting that something might be wrong. This is for a number of reasons, including the fact that even today it is still usually the mother who has the most contact with the children. She's often the one who chauffeurs them to and from extracurricular activities, takes them to doctor's appointments, talks with their teachers over the phone when the need arises, develops a relationship with the school, and spends the most time with them. It's not surprising then that Mom is the one who relays messages to Dad regarding the children—she is the bearer of ill tidings. Because Dad usually does not spend as much time with the children as does Mom, he is expected to accept something that he's not really sure about. It then becomes difficult for Dad to accept that his child is not one hundred percent perfect, because that is how he sees the child. Often, Dad has to work through his denial before the child can be treated.

Anger is common, as is grief. We have a right and a need to grieve—it is a legitimate response to the tremendous loss we feel. We grieve for our child, and we grieve for ourselves.

Assessing the Need for Professional Intervention

When a patient arrives in a hospital emergency room, an ER doctor gets whatever patient history she can as quickly as possible, either from the patient, family members, emergency crews, witnesses—whoever can give her the information she needs.

For example, a patient brought in by ambulance from an

auto accident may have several wounds that draw the doctor's eye, even though they might not be life threatening. However, the heart attack the patient was suffering before the crash might kill the patient if it goes unrecognized.

In assessing the need for professional help for your child, then, we can look first to those problems that can cause the child grievous injury, permanent disability, or death. For example, a threat to commit suicide should always be taken seriously, whatever the age of the person. The old saw that the person who threatens suicide is probably not sincere or that she is just crying out for help is not always true!

Although many adults who have threatened to commit suicide have made that threat to manipulate and control others and have no intention to harm themselves, children are not as likely to be "conning" others into compliance with their wishes by threatening suicide. (Of course, any threat to commit suicide—regardless of its motivation—should always be taken seriously.) Of equal concern is the fact that many completed suicides are apparently accidental—the person was merely threatening suicide to manipulate and control others. When that threat did not have the desired result, the person felt that if he just moved closer to actually doing it, the person he was trying to manipulate would save him or give in to his demands—but the would-be suicide was *accidentally* successful!

Young children, particularly, have no realistic understanding of the finality of death. Even teenagers may have romantic notions of being saved at the last moment by a caring other. Psychological autopsies of many suicides have revealed that often the person took an overdose of, for example, sleeping pills approximately a half hour before she knew that a parent or spouse would be coming home from work. The tragedy comes when the unplanned-for accident, a mechanical breakdown, or simply a change in plans prevents the savior from arriving for hours or days. Any threat by a child to commit suicide should be treated as a medical emergency!

Unless you are willing to bet your child's life on your ability to discern that he's merely trying to manipulate or that an attempt at manipulation won't accidentally result in a completed suicide, you're well advised to take the child immediately to the nearest medical facility. The emergency room of a psychiatric hospital is preferred, but any hospital ER is satisfactory.

The point is that any time that you feel you are witnessing an indication that your child is planning to harm herself, you must take immediate action. Some indications, taken together but rarely individually, might be the following:

- Recent loss of interest in activities that always attracted your child before

- Planning to or actually giving away toys or other possessions that your child has treasured

- Comments such as "Life is a drag," "Life is not worth living," "I wonder what it's like to be dead?" and "I'm just no good"

- Sudden noticeable worsening in personal hygiene

- Change in sleep habits, either from needing little sleep to sleeping all the time, or from sleeping well to sleeping poorly or hardly at all

- Marked difference in eating habits

- Any comments or behavior that indicates that your child is not planning on future activities—on not having a future

- Loss of interest in school, grades, social events, friends

The alert and knowledgeable parent reading this section will recognize that a number of these red flags are also indicators of depression. Even if the number of these indicators and their severity don't add up to potential suicide in your mind, more than one or two should alert you to the strong likelihood that your child may be depressed. Whether you're concerned about potential suicide or depression, exhibiting a number of these signals is a strong indication that your child should be evaluated by a mental health professional.

Some situations demand the immediate involvement of a mental health professional either because the child has instant, emergent needs, or because long-term damage or loss is likely if the child is not treated right away. Some other medical emergencies include the following:

- Substance abuse-induced behavior (delusions, hallucinations)

- Aggressive behavior toward others, either physical violence or verbal threats

- Self-injurious behaviors (intentional cutting or burning of self)

- Out-of-control behavior (temper tantrums of abnormal duration or intensity)

- Clearly irrational behavior (such as walking into the path of oncoming vehicles with no apparent awareness of danger)

- Extreme excitement clearly out of proportion to the situation (manic behavior)

Although the need to seek professional help for your child's emotional problems will not always constitute a medical emergency, other problems—less dramatic but important to the quality of your child's life—also demand prompt attention. Although these problems may not seem as urgent as those that can kill your child, ignore them at your child's peril, because they can mean the difference between a healthy, effective, and happy life and a mean existence devoid of satisfaction, pleasure, and love.

Listening to Your Child

Listening is the most important tool you can use as a parent when trying to assess the seriousness of your child's problem and whether the help of a professional is warranted. Sometimes, the concerns that your child voices will parallel your own, and you may be tempted to talk with her about her problems as you would another adult; after all, she has similar concerns, right? Resist that urge! No matter how logical it may seem to you to discuss your child's problems with her from an adult perspective, you must remember that your child is a *child* and not merely a younger, shorter version of an adult.

Instead of hearing the opening phrases of your child's problem, forming an immediate opinion of what the trouble is, and providing a solution, just sit quietly and really *listen* to your child. Nod appreciatively as you hear a point she is making; show that you really do understand. Question, gently and with tact, those things you don't understand; let her feel that you are committed to hearing her, really understanding. Watch her face carefully; observe how she holds her body, uses her hands to help express herself. With careful listening and skilled observation, you can begin to understand what's important to her and what she is actually telling you.

When looking at your child's fears and worries, it's important to keep in mind the significance they hold for your child. Never demean his concerns; instead, acknowledge that you understand their importance to him. Being available to your child, being prepared to spend time hearing what he has to say, acknowledging the child's right to have concerns, and taking them seriously may be all you ever need to do to help him handle the challenges of his life.

Many of the difficulties your child may be having will resolve themselves with time and experience, just as a cold tends to get better within a week or so whether you do anything for it or not. And, just as when your child has a cold, your obvious concern and empathy may well make the time between now and feeling better pass more quickly and less painfully.

Sometimes, though, helping a child resolve emotional turmoil takes more than a sympathetic ear and some chicken soup. Occasionally in the life of even the most emotionally healthy child, issues will take more than our concern and empathy to resolve. It's then when our ability to relate to our children is most seriously tested.

Even then, whether to call in a mental health professional or handle it ourselves is not a clear-cut decision. Sometimes, our ability to deal effectively with our children's concerns is compromised by our own discomfort in dealing with the concerns. Many parents are uncomfortable discussing, for example, masturbation. Others can handle discussions like this with imperturbability.

In situations like these, community resources can be an effective alternative. Many churches and synagogues maintain teen crisis lines to discuss sensitive topics with teens who are too embarrassed to discuss them with parents. Some of these houses of worship have established homework helplines for younger children, as well as crisis facilities for troubled children.

Whether to encourage or discourage your child from using such resources is a matter of personal preference. It's important to remember that information lines or crisis lines maintained by churches and synagogues will answer your child's questions, but almost always will slant their answers to conform with that particular faith's moral convictions on that question. For example, one church's information will address masturbation as a normal and healthy expression of the sexuality of young people, whereas another may condemn the practice as sinful. Before suggesting that your child call one of these crisis lines, it's important that you agree with the perspective that the church will probably take on such issues.

Schools, too, often offer counseling services for their students or centralized services for the school district's children. More secular than the church-sponsored services, they also will frequently address problems common to children. Before using these services, however, it's important to learn what stance they take on the concerns your child is likely to bring up and to assure yourself that you can live with their recommendations.

More involved or serious difficulties will take more comprehensive attention. Finding an appropriate mental health professional to work with your child's concerns is dealt with in more detail in chapter nine. For now, several suggestions are mentioned briefly to help you realize that personal resources need not be a block to receiving help for your child.

County mental health facilities. Across the United States, most counties maintain some type of county-funded mental health facility. These can range from full-blown mental hospitals in larger cities to part-time clinics in more rural settings. Regardless of the amount and nature of help provided, almost all county facilities can refer you to private providers as well as to other county, local, and state facilities where you may obtain help.

Medical school clinics. If you're fortunate enough to live near a medical school, it's likely that the department of psychiatry has an outpatient clinic for children. Often staffed by third- or fourth-year medical students or resident physicians in psychiatric training, such clinics always have fully trained, competent staff.

University graduate school clinics. Whether or not a medical school is nearby, major universities often are within driving distance. Graduate schools of psychology or social work often have clinics to see children and adults. As in medical school clinics, most of the work is performed by psychology and social work interns as part of their training. Most are very competent, and all are supervised by fully competent, licensed faculty.

PART II

Educating Yourself: Understanding Childhood Problems

FOUR

Childhood Disorders You Should Know About

E ach life stage that our children grow through on the way to becoming successful adults—from infancy through the teen years—has developmental milestones. Developmental milestones are the ages at which the majority of children have achieved certain developmental tasks. It is important to remember that these are averages. Your child may be somewhat behind or ahead of the schedule without great significance. If a child has a developmental disorder, the rate of learning and retention of important information may be inadequate for that child to ever acquire the self-care, social behavior, and thinking skills needed for independent living. Delays in achieving developmental milestones may well be within the range of normal variation, and most are. But at the other end of the spectrum, they may herald the presence of mental retardation or autism.

Developmental Disorders

The *Diagnostic and Statistical Manual of Mental Disorders, Fourth Edition (DSM-IV)* is the book often referred to as "the psychiatrist's bible." Published by the American Psychiatric Association in Washington, DC, the book is referred to often during the workday by psychiatrists, psychologists, and in fact, by all mental health professionals. Aside from its extraordinary value as an educational tool, its primary value to the mental health professional is as a resource to help determine the appropriate diagnosis for the conditions presented by patients and clients.

It is a compendium of the official consensus on what constitutes a psychiatric diagnostic entity, as well as of appropriate diagnostic criteria for each of the many diagnoses. The term *developmental disorder*, although not an official designation used in *DSM-IV*, is frequently used by those who work closely with children. Used by professionals most often when referring to mental retardation, learning disorders, and pervasive developmental disorders (PDDs), we use it similarly here. To better understand why these are called developmental disorders, it's helpful to note that mental retardation (MR), learning disorders (LDs), and PDDs are all listed in the *DSM-IV* under the heading, "Disorders Usually First Diagnosed in Infancy, Childhood, and Adolescence."

Although the term *developmental disorders* can always mean at least MR, LD, and PDD, it also may imply motor skills disorder, communication disorders, attention deficit and disruptive behaviors disorders, feeding and eating disorders of infancy or early childhood, tic disorders, elimination disorders, and others. You may observe in your child certain behaviors and activities or the failure to achieve expected developmental milestones. Either of these situations may imply a condition that warrants evaluation. We've listed each of these developmental disorders next, along with their most important signs and symptoms.

Mental Retardation

Developmentally delayed is another term used to describe mentally retarded children—children who, for one reason or another, do not develop age-appropriate cognitive skills. The children are seriously delayed or compromised in their capacity for problem-solving, thinking, and learning. As a result, they do not achieve the academic and social skills, nor the level of independence, that their peers enjoy. A range of one to three percent of children is believed to be within this group. Depending on the severity of their difficulties, these children usually test at an IQ of 70 or less on standard tests of intelligence.

There are four degrees of severity for mental retardation: mild, IQ level 50 to 70; moderate, IQ level 35 to 55; severe, IQ level 20 to 40; profound, IQ level below 20.

Important signs and symptoms include the following:

- The child appears to have significant difficulty learning new words, concepts, and behaviors, and is significantly behind peers in accomplishment. If IQ testing is done on a child old enough for formal testing, his score is approximately seventy or less. Your subjective sense that the infant or toddler is "slow" compared to children of the same age warrants an immediate call to the child's pediatrician.

- The child has noticeably more difficulty performing effectively compared to others of his age in two or more of the following areas: communication, self-care, social and interpersonal skills, use of community resources, self-direction, functional academic skills, work, leisure, health, and safety.

Pervasive Developmental Disorders

The pervasive developmental disorders (PDD) are a group of fairly rare conditions. Autism is the one disorder in the group that most laypeople have heard of, though the group also includes Rett's disorder, childhood disintegrative disorder (CDD), and Asperger's disorder (perhaps better known as Asperger's syndrome). Although there are significant differences in these disorders, children with autism and Asperger's disorder seem to have a much better life course than children with Rett's disorder or childhood disintegrative disorder. All four disorders are fairly rare, with autism being the most common. Even though these disorders are not common, they are significant because of the devastation they cause the individual and his family, especially with Rett's and CDD. Even though they are uncommon, more is known and understood about autism and Asperger's disorder than the others.

Autism
Children with autism are loners, shunning cooperative play and preferring solitary pursuits. Stereotypy, or the development of repetitive behaviors and rituals, is a hallmark of the disorder, frequently seen as head-banging or rocking. They tend not to be "cuddlers" and are likely to loudly reject any attempts to hold them close; eye-to-eye contact is limited or nonexistent.

Creative activity is usually restricted or even absent. Because language skills are often limited and always grossly delayed, these children frequently are hard to engage in meaningful conversation. Autistic children often relate to others in a manner similar to their relationship with the furniture in a room, appearing and behaving totally bereft of emotion at times. A failure to establish a significant bond with primary or other caretakers is commonly seen, making this a particularly disheartening disorder for parents.

Like mental retardation, autism is a very complex disorder; its origin is unclear, and its treatment is difficult. The most optimistic outcome occurs with early recognition and intervention.

Important signs and symptoms include the following:

- Difficulty in social interactions: problems looking others in the eye, "flat" or inappropriate facial expression, unusual body postures, and a lack of "body language" in social situations

- Doesn't develop friendships like others his age

- Never seems to go out of his way to share his interest in or excitement about anything, including his accomplishments

- Doesn't respond emotionally when spoken to or when interacting with others ("Like talking to a wall")

- Problems in communications, for example, a delay in or lack of development of spoken language, especially if he doesn't gesture or mime to help others understand him

- Even if he can speak adequately, shows no interest (or poor ability) in starting a conversation, or keeping one going

- Often uses the same words frequently or often uses his own made-up words

- Rarely involved in make-believe or fantasy play; isn't likely to pretend to be someone else (in play), such as in "Cops and Robbers"

- Has few interests; his behaviors and activities are often repetitive and stereotyped; you may see great preoccupation with only one or a few interests, that may seem odd or unusual to you, especially for the amount of focus or intensity put into them

- Rigidly adheres to specific routines or rituals that seem to accomplish nothing

• Performs some movement repetitively (for example, hand or finger flapping or even more complex body motions) and almost exactly the same way each time

• A strong and consistent interest in a part of a thing rather than the thing itself (special emphasis on one syllable in a word, not on the whole word itself; fascination with the "color" control on the TV remote, rather than on the remote in general or the TV as a whole)

• You notice before he's three years old that he seems far behind other children his age in the way he interacts with others socially; his use of language in communicating with others is delayed or abnormal; he rarely or never plays with toys (or uses other objects to represent toys or other things) or plays "pretend"

Understand that this long list of signs represents all the diagnostic criteria you could see in an autistic child. To make the diagnosis using *DSM-IV* would take a combination of *some* of the signs, not *all* of them.

Asperger's

To a hasty and superficial observer, Asperger's disorder (syndrome) would probably appear to be a minor subset of autism. Even though it's clear to most researchers that Asperger's must have a place close to autism on the spectrum of disorders, there are significant differences. Its essential features are shared with autism: severe and enduring impairment in social interaction and the development and consistent maintenance of just a small number of interests, behaviors, and activities that varies little over time. This disorder will cause substantial impairment in the child's ability to function in social, school, or other activities.

However, it is quite different from autism in two significant ways. Children with Asperger's show no major or clinically important delays in language development. Further, children with Asperger's are essentially normal with respect to cognitive development, curiosity about their environment, and developing age-appropriate skills for self-help. The ability to adapt to changing situations in their world also grows except in the area of social interactions, where they remain stilted, almost inanimate at times. Asperger's also seems to emerge later than autism; at least it appears to be recognized later. Motor delays or clumsiness may be noticed prior to the child's starting school. The child's problems with effective social interaction usually become more apparent after he starts school, with its continuously increasing demand for social facility. It's also common for the child's unusual or limited range of interests to emerge early in the school course, or at least to be recognized then. Children with Asperger's may seem cold at times and unable to empathize; that course usually continues in adulthood. But the potential for fully independent living is higher in Asperger's than in others of the PDD group.

Important signs and symptoms include:

- Little or no use of nonverbal communications, such as eye-to-eye gaze, gestures, changes in posture, and facial expression to facilitate social interaction

- Doesn't make friends like others at his developmental stage

- Does not seek out others to share in his interests, achievements, or "fun times"

- Repetitive and almost identical patterns of behaviors, interests, and anxieties shown in the following:

  - Complete preoccupation with one or more restricted but intricate patterns of interest that others perceive as abnormal in focus or intensity

  - Seemingly fixed adherence to specific but nonfunctional routines or rituals

  - Repetitive movements of hands, fingers, or whole body

  - Consistent preoccupation with parts of a thing rather than with the thing itself

  - No significant delay in acquiring language skills

  - No significant delay in developing thinking and reasoning or in developing age-appropriate curiosity about his environment, self-help skills, or ability to adapt to changing circumstances, except in her ability to relate effectively with others

As in autism, not all of the signs listed need to be met for diagnosis.

Other PDDs

Two other conditions are classified as pervasive developmental disorders: Rett's disorder and childhood disintegrative disorder (CDD). Rett's disorder is fairly rare, occurring much less frequently than autism. Epidemiological data are limited, but childhood disintegrative disorder also appears to be very rare.

We include these two disorders here because the earlier an accurate diagnosis is reached, the sooner the child can receive the care needed. Equally important, the parents of such a child will be spared perhaps years of frustration, pain, and struggle. Even though the statistical view would make the numbers seem trivial, receiving any of these diagnoses for one's child is anything but trivial.

In some ways, Rett's disorder and CDD are more insidious than either autism or Asperger's disorder. Both characteristically have periods of apparently normal growth and development prior to the onset of a serious deterioration of mental status and ability. The specific deficits associated with each disorder are different, but the prognosis with either is not encouraging.

With Rett's disorder there is apparently normal prenatal and perinatal development, with what seems like normal psychomotor development through the first five months after birth. There is also normal head circumference at birth. However, between five and forty-eight months after birth, head growth decelerates. Previously acquired purposeful hand skills are lost, and a hand-wringing or hand-washing movement develops. The child loses interest in social engagement and begins to show poorly coordinated gait or trunk movements. Development of language abilities becomes severely impaired in both the expressive and receptive components, and a severe psychomotor retardation develops. To date, Rett's has been reported only in females.

Childhood disintegrative disorder is frequently associated with severe mental retardation. Abnormal EEG studies (abnormal brain-wave test results) or evidence of a seizure disorder is more likely than in the other PDDs. It seems likely that the disorder results from some insult to the developing nervous system, though no specific mechanism has been identified. Occasionally, CDD is seen in association with another medical condition that could explain the developmental regression. Far more frequently, extensive investigation is not able to reveal a cause. There is apparently normal development for the first two years of life. Usually after age two, but before age ten, these children lose a significant amount of previously acquired skills in at least two of the five following areas:

- Language; expressive or receptive

- Adaptive behavior/social skills

- Bladder and/or bowel control

- Play activities

- Motor skills

They also show at least two of the following:

- Impairment in the quality of social interaction (lack of emotional reciprocity, failure to develop friendships)

- Impairment in the quality of communications (lack or delay of spoken language, inability to initiate or maintain a conversation, restricted vocabulary, lack of make-believe play)

- Patterns of behavior restricted and repetitive, as are activities, interests, and mannerisms

- The child's difficulties are not better explained by another specific PDD or by schizophrenia

Specific Developmental Disorders

We refer here to those developmental disorders other than MR and PDDs that interfere with normal intellectual, emotional, and physical development. Some of the disorders that fall under this heading are clearly learning disorders (LDs); their names and the focus of their pathology make that clear. Perhaps not as clear, but just as important to recognize, is that the other disorders listed in this section are also LDs. The way they impair learning and growth intellectually and emotionally may not be as direct, but their effect is to impede a child's progress as he struggles to succeed at learning.

All the disorders that follow, regardless of their immediate focus, impair learning in a basic and significant way.

Learning Disorders

DSM-IV establishes three basic learning disorders: reading disorder, mathematics disorder, and disorder of written expression.

These are specific entities, each causing an impairment of learning specific to its name. A fourth, learning disorder not otherwise specified, is sort of a catch basin for any other disorders that compromise learning but that do not meet the criteria for diagnosis of the other three.

Estimations of the prevalence of learning disorders depends on the agency making the determination and on the definitions it is using, but generally, two to ten percent is an accepted figure. According to the *DSM-IV*, approximately five percent of students in American schools are identified as being learning disordered.

Reading Disorder

Reading disorder is often popularly referred to as *dyslexia*. Most people commonly associate dyslexia with letter reversal when reading. Of course, children may exhibit many other difficulties with reading. When the *DSM-IV* officially changed the term for what used to be called *developmental reading disorder* to *reading disorder*, it made clear that the reading difficulties associated with dyslexia, as well as other difficulties with reading, were all to be encompassed by the new term.

Reading disorder can be one of the most problematic learning disorders, because the ability to read is basic to the ability to learn in our culture. Early detection of this disorder is essential; identification of the problem is, by itself, somewhat remedial. Reading achievement is the ability affected by this disorder, as seen in the child's competence in reading accuracy, comprehension, and speed. In a child with a reading disorder, measures of these indices will show achievement below predicted values for the child's age, measured intelligence, and level of education. This child will also experience significant interference with academic performance or in the performance of activities of daily living that require the ability to read. If sensory deficit exists (for example, poor eyesight, even when corrected), the reading problems exceed those usually associated with the deficit.

Unfortunately, mathematics disorder and disorder of written expression are often found in association with reading disorder. In fact, it's unusual to find either of these other disorders in the absence of reading disorder. Studies used in the United States may fail to carefully separate reading disorder from mathematics disorder and disorders of written expression, instead focusing on learning disorders generally. Even so, four percent of school-aged children in the United States are believed to have reading disorder.

Important signs and symptoms include:

- Reading achievement is substantially below the level expected for the child's age, intelligence, and academic level (grade)

- Significant problems with academic achievement or with any tasks that require the ability to read

- If there are sensory deficits (poor eyesight, for instance), the reading problem is greater than would be expected with the deficit alone

Mathematics Disorder

As in reading disorder, the primary feature of mathematics disorder is achievement that falls substantially below that predicted by the child's age, measured intelligence, and academic level. This disorder significantly interferes with the child's performance academically, and with other activities that require mathematical skills. If a sensory deficit (problems with vision, hearing, etc.) is noted, the problems in mathematics that the child encounters are significantly greater than would normally be associated with the deficit. As in reading disorder, a number of areas of mental activity can be affected. However, they are more specifically enumerated by the *DSM-IV* in this classification. For example, it mentions "linguistic" skills (where a child might have trouble understanding mathematical symbols), "perceptual" skills (difficulty in reading or recognizing mathematical symbols or arithmetic signs), "mathematical" skills (counting objects, following a sequence of operations, etc.), as well as some others. It is estimated that one percent of school-aged children in the United States have mathematical disorder.

Important signs and symptoms include:

- Mathematical achievement is substantially below the level expected for the child's age, intelligence, and academic level (grade)

- Significant problems with academic achievement and with any tasks that require mathematical ability

- If there are sensory deficits (poor eyesight or hearing), the

mathematical problem is greater than would be expected
with the deficit alone

Disorder of Written Expression

This disorder causes difficulties in writing skills. Although poor
handwriting is not a necessary component of this disorder, it is
often seen along with more substantial problems. The child may,
for example, evidence problems with writing skills by many
grammatical or spelling errors, poor paragraph organization, and
excessively poor handwriting. If there are any sensory deficits,
the problems with writing skills are notably worse than would be
expected with the deficits alone. Here, as in the other learning
disorders, there is the likelihood that a number of difficulties are
combining to cause problems with the child's ability to compose
written text. Making the diagnosis of this disorder may involve
examination of an extensive collection of the child's writing,
comparing it in quality with that of other children of comparable
age, intellect, and grade level. This disorder is commonly associated with other learning disorders.

Important signs and symptoms include:

- Quality of written expression is substantially below the
  level expected for the child's age, intelligence, and academic level (grade)

- The problem with writing skills causes significant problems
  with academic achievement and with any tasks that
  require the ability to write

- If there are sensory deficits (poor eyesight or hearing), the
  problem with writing is greater than would be expected
  with the deficit alone

As we address the remaining seven diagnostic groups, please
keep in mind that, although these disorders are not explicitly
called learning disorders, we believe that most are. Simply put, if
the disorder can significantly interfere with the ability of the
child to learn and to grow into an effective and independent
adult, we consider it a learning disorder.

Communication Disorders

Language is the use of words to communicate a specific meaning
to others. Disorders of language can limit a child's ability to com-

municate effectively and can impair her capacity for learning. Because a child's early years are so important as a foundation for future learning in both academic and social skills, disorders of language acquisition and use need to be detected early and treated immediately.

Although delayed speech deserves evaluation, parents need to keep in mind that delayed speech alone is not necessarily pathological. Some children are simply more verbal, whereas others may not start to speak until age two. As long as no pathology is associated with a delay, children who start speaking later than others show no long-term deficit and catch up to their earlier-speaking peers rapidly.

Problems with syntax or word use may reflect serious cognitive difficulties or may be related to a more slowly, but still normally maturing, nervous system. Because both receptive speech and expressive speech are important to a child's normal development, difficulties in either should be evaluated if they do not correct themselves quickly. Inasmuch as early speech problems are fairly common, an evaluation might reveal no serious problem. Nevertheless, because problems with speech can be so damaging to a child's development, they should be investigated.

Articulation problems concern a child's difficulty with physically saying words clearly and understandably. Here, too, a normally but slowly developing nervous system may be the cause. Because both emotional and physical problems can contribute to these difficulties, however, it is wise to have an evaluation done.

This group consists of four primary communications disorders (expressive language disorder, mixed receptive-expressive language disorder, phonological disorder, and stuttering). A fifth, communication disorder not otherwise specified (NOS), is the catch basin for the group, into which are placed problems that clearly are communication based but that don't fit the exact criteria for any of the four primary disorders. In the four primary diagnoses, provision is made for inclusion of physiological causes if present and determined. However, none requires a clear understanding of the cause for the diagnosis to be made. The primary thrust of diagnosis in this group is to describe and document whatever interference there is with the child's academic, occupational, or social communication. Often, psychiatrists and other therapists can help children make great strides in overcoming the greatest limitations that these disorders can cause. Where the psychiatric diagnosis has a general medical or neurological aspect, these mental health professionals can be of great assistance to other physicians and clinicians who will work with the physiological aspect. When psychiatric attention is combined with that of other specialties as needed, the child has the greatest opportunity to overcome the disorder, if that's possible, or to learn to accommodate it with the least possible interference with his quality of life.

It is likely that the primary disorders have a neurological component in many cases. Even so, not infrequently, no determination of neurological pathology is ever made. Although each individual must be considered independently, it is probably fair to say that each affected individual has an emotional/psychological component to his disorder. The emotional/psychological component represents either part of the etiology of the disorder or an almost unavoidable result of having it. Many of the symptoms of this group of disorders represent fertile soil for embarrassment and shame to grow in the affected child. The (perhaps) inadvertent cruelty of other youngsters toward a child who is "different" causes much unnecessary suffering. For children with developmental disorders, beyond the threat of immediate trauma of insults and taunts from peers is the substantial potential for lifelong emotional and social disability. Initial evaluation of these disorders by both a neurologist and a psychiatrist is essential. Physicians of other specialties also may need to be part of the treatment team for these children. Most often allied health professionals, such as audiologists, speech pathologists, and so forth, will be necessary for the most effective treatment and the greatest reduction of symptoms.

Expressive Language Disorder

Disorders of language can limit the ability to communicate effectively and can impair capacity for learning. Language difficulties interfere with academic and occupational achievement and with social communication. Speech difficulties that occur with this disorder may include limitations on the types of sentences used, such as their length and complexity, difficulty in acquiring new words, limitations on the amount of speech, word-finding errors, limited vocabulary, and others. The psychosocial impact of this disorder without diagnosis and effective treatment can result in the individual being limited in educational, employment, and social contexts. Disorders of language acquisition and use need to be detected early and treated immediately.

Important signs and symptoms include:

• Testing substantially below measures of expressive language development as predicted by nonverbal intellectual testing and level of receptive language development

• Language difficulties become serious enough to interfere with academic and occupational accomplishment and with social communication

Mixed Receptive-Expressive Language Disorder

This disorder is similar to expressive language disorder. An individual with this disorder has the difficulties seen in the previously discussed disorder, with the addition of impairment in receptive language development. That is, she might have problems not only expressing herself with language but with understanding it. The further difficulties with receptive language are largely due to problems with auditory processing.

An important difference here is that detection of the receptive component might be much more difficult than detection of the expressive component. Although we can hear the expressive speech difficulties, we have to detect and correctly interpret the child's further problem, which often appears as the child's frequent misunderstanding of what she has been told, or as seeming disobedience in an otherwise compliant child. The subtle and more difficult to detect receptive components and the potential for serious learning and social consequences for the undiagnosed and untreated child make this an important and challenging disorder to treat.

In addition to the symptoms for expressive language disorder, signs include the following:

• The child frequently misunderstands what she has been told

• A usually compliant child frequently seems to disobey

Phonological Disorder

This disorder concerns the inability to use speech sounds that are appropriate to the individual's age and development. Errors and difficulty in appropriate speech sound production (for example, substitution of one sound for another or reversal of enunciated letter sounds) are frequent and may include sound distortions, sound substitutions, and sound omissions. Hearing impairment or neurological difficulties may or may not be present as clear causes.

Important signs and symptoms include the following:

- Inability to use speech sounds in a manner appropriate for age

- Speech sound production difficulties become serious enough to interfere with academic, occupational, and social development

Stuttering

With stuttering, both the time patterning and normal fluency of speech are inappropriate for the age of the speaker. It can be characterized by prolongations of sounds or syllables, frequent repetitions, and other disarticulations. These difficulties interfere with the individual's academic or occupational achievement and with his social communication. With a disorder that is variable in presentation, the severity often changes with the social context. It is usually exacerbated in stressful social situations, while it may be absent when reading aloud, singing, and other situations. Stuttering can be accompanied by various motor activities that are strongly suggestive of tics, often involving the eyes, lips, face, and head movements. Onset is insidious, beginning most often between two and seven years of age and before age ten in ninety-eight percent of cases. The emotional and psychological effect on the child who stutters can be powerful. Research suggests that up to eighty percent of individuals with stuttering recover. Perhaps as many as sixty percent recover spontaneously, typically before age sixteen. The long-term harm, however, could easily continue after the stuttering ceases.

As youngsters, we've all known children who stuttered—a classmate, a cousin, a fellow church member. And we all can remember the ridicule and scorn some children inflicted on that individual. Even though the child may recover from the stuttering in mid to late adolescence, the probability of his self-esteem and self-image having suffered is high. The social experiences of childhood set the tone for adolescence; the adolescent years are even more significant in setting the tone for one's ability as an adult to relate to others in a social and business context. Many who stuttered as children have matured with little or no apparent ill effect. Some, however, find that their social and occupational future is compromised by the low self-esteem and low self-image acquired as results of childhood stuttering.

Even though the statistical odds favor your child's recovery, we recommend that any child who develops a stutter be evaluated. If neurologic or other medical problems that could contribute to the stuttering can be ruled out, a referral to a good speech pathologist is available from most pediatric neurologists. If you believe that your child is experiencing emotional problems because of the stuttering (has become quiet and shy or seems anxious or depressed), request a referral to a mental health professional specializing in stuttering.

Important signs and symptoms include:

- The child demonstrates a disturbance in the time patterning and normal fluency of speech that is inappropriate for his age; disturbances can include pausing within a word, repeating sounds or syllables, leaving unfilled pauses in speech or pauses filled with nonword sounds, prolonging sounds, and speaking whole-word, monosyllabic repetitions ("There h-h-h-he goes!") and interjections; may avoid problem words by using word substitution and may speak words with excessive physical tension

- The fluency difficulties interfere with academic or occupational success and social communication

- If a sensory deficit or a speech-motor problem is present, the child's difficulties with speech are greater than those expected from these problems alone

Motor Skills Disorder

This is the smallest of the groups of disorders that we consider in this area; it consists of only one illness: developmental coordination disorder (DCD). The defining feature of this disorder is a marked impairment of the development of motor coordination. For a child to be diagnosed with DCD, the disorder must interfere significantly with the child's academic performance and success or with daily living.

This disorder manifests itself differently with age and development. For example, a young child may appear clumsy and be delayed in achieving motor developmental milestones such as sitting, crawling, walking, et cetera. Older children will display difficulty with crafts, playing ball, handwriting, and other tasks requiring dexterity and coordination. One or more of the communications disorders is often associated with this disorder, but this association is not one of the diagnostic criteria. The course is variable; some children develop essentially normal coordination as they grow older. For some, the lack of coordination is lifelong.

Important signs and symptoms include:

- Daily activities requiring motor coordination are performed substantially below predicted ability in light of age and measured intelligence; this will be reflected by delays in achieving motor milestones

- The disorder significantly interferes with academic success or activities of daily living

- The problems are not due to a general medical condition (for instance, muscular dystrophy, cerebral palsy, or hemiplegia)

- When mental retardation is also present, the motor problems are greater than would be associated with mental retardation alone

ADHD

Much has been written in recent years about ADHD. Called many things over the last hundred years, it is now seen as a legitimate and treatable clinical entity. Even so, most of the traits of ADHD are seen in many children who do not have this disorder. What separates the children who do from the children who don't?

The three cardinal traits of ADHD are impulsivity, distractibility, and hyperactivity. This definition is perplexing to some parents, because almost all children display some or all of these traits at one time or another. The differentiating factors are whether the traits are pervasive in the child and the degree to which they are present. Many young children are occasionally impulsive, but there is usually some awareness of the outside world even in their impulsive state. The child with ADHD is impulsive most of the time—behaving as if he is oblivious to the real world and unaware that impulsive acts might have negative consequences.

Some children display distractibility in that they can maintain their attention on a certain toy or activity for only a comparatively short time. At other times and in different circumstances, they're not distractible. Unless totally absorbed in the task at hand, children with ADHD are often constantly and easily distracted, finding it difficult if not impossible to remain on task—even when they want to.

Many children, especially preschool children, are said to be *hyperactive*. Usually the term is misused to denote an active, busy child—one often in constant motion. The child with ADHD, however, displays a different quality in her peripatetic, almost frenetic activity. Whereas a child without ADHD may run into her room, emptying her toy chest in seemingly pointless activity, they may merely be searching for a specific toy, albeit in "fast mode." Though not immediately apparent, there is purpose to her hurried activity. A child with ADHD might well run into her room, flinging about toys from her toy chest in a similar way, but close observation will not yield any apparent motive. Her hyperactive behavior often lacks purpose, being haphazard and pointless.

Because of its importance and its prevalence in the United States today, more information specific to ADHD and how it can affect school performance is discussed in chapter six. However, for consistency and easy use, we include some important data about diagnosis:

- The child must display at least six symptoms of a list specific to inattention:

  - Typically, is careless or doesn't give close attention to schoolwork, activities, or other work

  - Finds sustaining attention difficult during activities

  - Does not appear to listen when addressed directly

  - Often fails to follow instructions accurately or to finish assignments, whether in schoolwork or home chores

  - Frequently has difficulty in organization

- Often dislikes and attempts to avoid tasks requiring continuous, sustained attention

- Frequently misplaces objects needed to complete tasks

- Easily distracted

- Forgetful in daily activities

OR

- The child needs to display at least six symptoms of a list specific to *hyperactivity-impulsivity*

  Hyperactivity:

  - Frequently squirms in seat or fidgets with hands or feet

  - Fails to remain seated in situations in which it is expected

  - Climbs and runs in inappropriate situations (adolescents may simply feel restless)

  - Frequently cannot play or be at leisure quietly

  - Frequently chatters on

  Impulsivity:

  - Frequently doesn't wait for questions to be finished, instead blurts out answer

  - Waiting for his turn in a group situation is difficult

  - Frequently interrupts others

- Either some inattentive symptoms or some hyperactive-impulsive symptoms must have been present before seven years of age and must have caused impairment

- Clinically significant impairment in at least two settings (academic, social, or occupational) must be clearly evident

The following are the three primary ADHD disorders:

- Attention deficit hyperactivity disorder, combined type

- Attention deficit hyperactivity disorder, predominantly inattentive type (has at least six of the "inattentive" symptoms)

- Attention deficit hyperactivity disorder, predominantly hyperactive-impulsive type (has at least six of the "hyperactive-impulsive" symptoms)

Oppositional Defiant Disorder and Conduct Disorder

Although the important considerations that define ODD are not identical to those of conduct disorder (CD), they are of identical genre; the essential differences lie only in the seriousness of offenses committed and the disdain held for the rules of society. Oppositional defiant disorder is the milder of the two.

Most adolescents diagnosed with CD were previously diagnosed with ODD. Of the adolescents adjudicated "juvenile delinquents," the vast majority carry the CD diagnosis or meet the criteria for that diagnosis; many had previously qualified as ODD. CD would be an appropriate diagnostic consideration for the high school junior who often threatens and intimidates others or who is caught rifling through his classmates' lockers during fifth period.

Oppositional Defiant Disorder

In this disorder, behavior and attitude define the problem. The most important feature of ODD is a recurring pattern of defiant, hostile, negativistic, and disobedient behavior toward authority figures lasting at least six months. Eight target behaviors cited in *DSM-IV* describe how the child acts. These include arguing with adults, actively defying or refusing to comply with adult requests or rules, and being spiteful or vindictive, among others. The rest are similar in nature, stressing disobedience and disregard for rules, refusal to take responsibility for one's acts, and deliberately annoying others.

The child who is diagnosed with this disorder behaves in this fashion more frequently than do others of comparable age and developmental level. These behaviors must lead to significant interference at home, in school, or in social activities. Unwillingness to cooperate, negotiate, or "give in" are hallmark traits of this disorder. ODD usually becomes evident prior to age eight, and its development is typically gradual, first appearing at school, then worsening and appearing at home and in other settings. Unfortunately, if not recognized and dealt with effectively, it is often a developmental precursor to conduct disorder (CD).

Certain family milieus tend to aid the development of this disorder. For instance, it is more common in families with great marital discord. It is also seen more frequently in families in which at least one parent has a history of a mood disorder, ADHD, antisocial personality disorder, or other psychiatric condition.

ODD is also a "frequent flyer" with many other disorders seen in children; that is, it is often a *comorbidity* (a simultaneously occurring disorder). Particularly evident when present with ADHD, Asperger's disorder, OCD, and mood and anxiety disorders, especially depression, it may be present only subtly with other disorders, though its contribution to pathology in that child may be significant.

As serious as this disorder can be, it usually does not include acts of violence or some of the other overtly antisocial characteristics of conduct disorder. Untreated, however, there is a good chance that the child with ODD will go on to develop conduct disorder. If you think your child fits the criteria, it's important that you arrange for an evaluation as soon as possible.

Here is some important information regarding diagnosis:

- The child demonstrates a pattern of behavior that is hostile, negative, and defiant for at least six months, during which at least four of the behaviors mentioned (from a list of eight behaviors) are present; these count as meeting the criteria only if the behavior is exhibited more frequently than in other children of similar age and developmental level

- The behavior problems cause a significant disturbance in academic, social, or familial settings

- The behaviors must not be present only during a psychotic or mood disorder

Conduct Disorder

Although all the disorders discussed here are serious in one way or another, conduct disorder is one of the few in which physical harm to others is a realistic concern. The pattern central to the disorder is the exhibition of persistent and repetitive behaviors that can include rule breaking, a disregard for the basic rights of others, and flouting of age-appropriate societal norms. Behaviors are grouped into four main categories: aggressive, in which the individual threatens or actually harms people or animals; nonaggressive, in which property damage replaces human injury; deceitfulness or theft; and serious violations of rules. The behavior must significantly interfere with academic, occupational, or social functioning. Most often, the child or teenager is seen by adults and peers as delinquent or "bad," rather than mentally ill.

Aggressive behavior toward others is commonly seen with this disorder, including bullying, intimidation, the use or display of weapons, and even rape or homicide. Deliberately destroying the property of others is also common; arson is often used as a means to destroy. Breaking and entering, lying to and cheating others, and stealing without confrontation are fairly common among adolescents with this disorder. The two subtypes, childhood onset and adolescent onset, differ most significantly in that childhood onset manifests symptoms of the disorder prior to ten years of age, and adolescent onset doesn't manifest symptoms of the disorder until after age ten. Behaviorally, a child with adolescent onset CD tends to be less violent and aggressive and is also less likely to have persistent conduct disorder. They also develop adult antisocial personality disorder less frequently.

This disorder also has severity specifiers: mild, moderate, and severe, depending on the range and severity of the offenses committed. Not surprisingly, males are much more frequently diagnosed with this disorder than are females. Treatment usually includes both behavior therapy and psychotherapy. This disorder is fairly complex, and treatment most likely will not be brief; developing new life habits takes time. Often, medication is added to the therapeutic regimen, especially if there are difficulties with attention or depression, which are likely. Effective treatment offers the best chance these children have for improvement.

Important information regarding diagnosis:

- There is evidence of three or more acts in the following categories:

    - Aggression toward people or animals

    - Destruction of property

    - Deceitfulness

    - Serious rule violation

- The behavior problems must have caused a significant impairment in function in academic, occupational, or social settings

- To be diagnosed after age eighteen, the individual cannot meet the criteria for antisocial personality disorder

Feeding and Eating Disorders of Infancy and Early Childhood

This group consists of three disorders that are relatively uncommon: pica, rumination disorder, and feeding disorder of infancy or early childhood. If your infant or toddler displays signs of any of these disorders, see your pediatrician.

Pica

Pica is the persistent eating of nonnutritive substances such as dirt, paint, clay, et cetera, for more than one month. The substances chosen to eat seem to vary with age and developmental level and usually come to medical attention only when there is an associated medical problem (poisoning, intestinal infections, or mechanical bowel problems, for example). In most cases, pica starts in infancy and usually remits within several months. It is, however, also associated with mental retardation and pervasive developmental disorder (PDD); the more severe the retardation, the higher the prevalence. It is important to note that pica does not, by itself, indicate either mental retardation or PDD. It is occasionally reported that a vitamin or mineral deficiency was noted in a pica patient; this is not the rule, however. Note, too, that in some cultures the eating of dirt is believed to be of some value. Before age eighteen to twenty-four months, mouthing and even eating nonfood items are not unusual. However, if your child displays this behavior after two years of age, talk with your child's pediatrician—he can evaluate your child and take appropriate action.

Rumination Disorder

This disorder occurs in a child after a period of normal functioning and consists of seemingly voluntary regurgitation. Usually there is continued chewing of the partially digested food, often with reswallowing, though with occasional ejection. Psychosocial difficulties that predispose may include inadequate stimulation, stressful situations, neglect, and ineffective parent-child relationships. This disorder can develop in the context of other developmental problems but can also occur in otherwise normal infants, remitting spontaneously. It usually begins at three to twelve months.

Parents who observe this behavior in their child are strongly urged to take their child to their pediatrician for an evaluation for several important reasons: The child may have congenital anomalies or other medical or surgical conditions that require immediate attention. If any of these other medical conditions exist, they must be corrected as soon as possible to afford the infant an opportunity for normal growth and development. The loss of weight or failure to gain weight that might accompany this disorder is an ominous sign and demands immediate medical attention. Otherwise, inadequate physical and intellectual development might occur. In serious cases of malnutrition caused by this disorder, or more likely by an underlying medical problem, death can occur, with mortality rates of up to twenty-five percent having been reported. Although this is not a medical emergency the first time it happens, if a pattern appears to be emerging, the child should be evaluated immediately.

Feeding Disorder of Infancy or Early Childhood

The most significant feature of this disorder is the continuing failure to eat adequately over a one-month period—resulting in the failure to gain weight or in a significant weight loss. This diagnosis cannot be made when there is a general medical condition present that is severe enough to explain a reluctance to eat, nor when symptoms can be better explained by another mental disorder. A wide range of parental difficulties can exist, from inappropriate feeding techniques to active psychopathology of the parent, though none of these need be present. Neurological problems and preexisting inadequate development can also be causes. Most commonly, onset of this disorder occurs in the first year of life, but it may not develop until two or three years of age. When it occurs at later ages, the developmental risk appears to be less.

Considering that some difficulties with eating and feeding are almost universal in infants, most parents are reluctant to become unduly alarmed over a short (two days to a week) period of poor appetite. However, malnutrition in severe cases can be life threatening, so the child should be evaluated immediately. Though the disorder described here may not exist in the child, she is medically deserving of an evaluation to rule it out or to discover any other general medical cause for her failure to thrive.

Tic Disorders

A tic is a sudden and repeated involuntary movement of a part of the body. Tics can occur in any part of the body but are most frequently seen in the face, hands, or legs. Many people with tics can prevent them or stop them for brief periods, but the effort can be enormous and unsustainable. A vocal tic is one in which the individual emits a grunt, groan, hiss, or other sound involuntarily. Usually these vocal tics are not comprised of coherent words, but in one special case they can be.

Transient tic disorders have been estimated to affect up to ten percent of early school-aged children. These transient tics usually fade and ultimately stop on their own. If a tic lasts more than one year, it is chronic. A special type of tic disorder called Tourette's disorder is discussed later.

Most types of tics can be controlled with medication. Often, tic disorders are seen in combination with other disorders, especially those involving attention, like ADHD, or others, like obsessive-compulsive disorder.

Tourette's Disorder

This is primarily a neurological disorder, characterized by involuntary movements, inappropriate words, and uncontrollable vocal sounds. Facial tics are usually the first manifestation, when the affected child may blink his eyes excessively, twitch his nose, or have facial contortions or grimaces. With progression, the child may also stretch his neck characteristically, stamp his feet, or twist his body. Part of the diagnostic criteria includes multiple motor tics, in fact. The criteria also call for vocal tics—the production of unnecessary and uncontrolled sounds. These sounds may be as simple as unnecessary but continuous throat clearing, cough, or sniff, or they might be a grunt, bark, or shout. Approximately ten percent of individuals with Tourette's disorder involuntarily shout obscenities (a phenomenon known as coprolalia). A small number constantly repeat the words of others (known as echolalia). Often associated with Tourette's disorder are obsessions and compulsions, sometimes as powerful as those associated with OCD. In fact, if these people did not have Tourette's disorder, but had the same level of obsessions and compulsions, many would qualify for a diagnosis of OCD.

Hyperactivity, distractibility, and impulsivity are also fairly common in these individuals, leading to the theory of a relationship between Tourette's and ADHD. Onset is usually during childhood or adolescence but can be as early as age two. It is defined as starting before eighteen years. Usually lifelong, it often has periods of remission lasting from weeks to years. Often, the disorder diminishes in severity and frequency during adolescence or by early adulthood. Sometimes the symptoms disappear completely, usually by early adulthood. Several times more prevalent in males than females, it occurs in approximately four to five individuals per ten thousand.

Important information regarding diagnosis:

- Though not necessarily concurrently, both multiple motor tics and vocal tics have been present at some time during the course of the illness

- For a child to qualify as having Tourette's disorder, the tics must occur many times a day, usually a group of them at a time, nearly every day for more than one year. There cannot be a tic-free period of more than three months

- The difficulties cause great distress or significantly impair social, occupational, or other important areas of function

- Onset must be before eighteen years old

- The condition is not caused by a substance (for instance, drugs or alcohol) or a general medical condition

Chronic Motor or Vocal Tic Disorder

The key feature of this disorder is either motor tics *or* vocal tics, but not both. Aside from this difference, the *DSM-IV* criteria are essentially the same as for Tourette's. Any difference would be in the severity of symptoms, with individuals with Tourette's showing greater impairment in function and more severe symptoms.

Important information regarding diagnosis:

• Either single or multiple motor tics or vocal tics have been present during the course of the illness

• The balance of the criteria is essentially the same as for Tourette's, except for these points:

  • The functional impairment is usually less than with Tourette's, which generally has more severe symptoms and greater functional impairment

  • The condition has never met the criteria for Tourette's disorder

Because both disorders can appear within the same family, Tourette's and chronic motor tic or vocal tic disorder are believed to be genetically related.

Elimination Disorders

These disorders can be very troublesome for both parent and child. Encopresis, repeated defecation into inappropriate places, is often socially isolating for the child—fear of an accident has stopped many overnights before they ever started. Similarly, enuresis—the repeated urination, during either day or night, into clothes or bedding—also may have a chilling effect on the social behavior of the children who have it.

Both disorders may involve involuntary or voluntary elimination. In both, the passage of feces or urine is most often involuntary, but occasionally may be voluntary. The child with either has a powerful tool to control his parents, though usually the elimination is not consciously willed.

The age of the child is an essential feature of these disorders; a chronological age of at least four years (or a mental age of at least four years, in the case of children with developmental delays) is necessary for encopresis. For a child to qualify for the diagnosis, the event must occur at least once a month for at least three months. Primary encopresis occurs when the child has never established continence; secondary encopresis is when the child develops this disturbance after having established continence. There are two subtypes. The first is with constipation and overflow incontinence. This occurs as a direct result of constipation. Poorly formed and loose stool leaks, often continuously, during the day and night. This tends to resolve with the effective treatment of the constipation. The second type is without constipation and overflow incontinence. There's no evidence of constipation, and the feces are generally normally formed and of proper consistency. Rather than continuous, soiling is intermittent. The deposition of stool is sometimes in a prominent, as well as inappropriate, location. Often this behavior is linked with oppositional defiant disorder or conduct disorder.

With enuresis, the child must have a chronological or mental age of at least five years. Here, the required frequency is at least twice a week for at least three months. Primary and secondary enuresis exist, as well. As with encopresis, primary enuresis is when the child has never been continent of urine; by definition, this begins at age five. Secondary enuresis is when the child has been continent of urine for a period of time, then becomes incontinent again. There are also three subtypes: nocturnal only, when the incontinence is only at night; diurnal only, when the incontinence is only during the daytime; and nocturnal and diurnal, a combination of the two previous subtypes.

Although both disorders frequently cause disturbances socially, academically, or in other important areas of function, the necessity for impairment in these areas is found only with enuresis. Of course, in neither disorder can the primary cause be a general medical condition or the result of medications or other substances (for example, laxatives or diuretics).

Important information regarding diagnosis of encopresis:

- Feces are repeatedly passed into inappropriate places (whether intentional or not)

- Incidents occur at least once a month for at least three months

- The child is at least four years of age chronologically or mentally

- Incidents are not due to a substance, such as a laxative, or a general medical condition; except that constipation may be involved

Important information regarding diagnosis of enuresis:

- Repeated urination, either involuntary or voluntary into clothes or bedding

- Incidents occur at least twice a week for three months and cause significant impairment or distress in social or academic functioning

- The child must be at least five years of age chronologically or the developmental equivalent

- The disorder cannot be a result of using a substance such as a diuretic, or of a general medical condition

When considering the presence of either disorder, it is important to keep in mind that a significant number of medical conditions cause either fecal or urinary incontinence and that the child may have no conscious intent. Similarly, many of the physical conditions that can cause encopresis or enuresis can have largely psychological origins. Children displaying symptoms of either disorder are deserving of immediate evaluation.

Other Disorders of Infancy, Childhood, or Adolescence

The disorders in this section are those that do not logically fit in any of the other categories, yet they are nonetheless considered disorders of infancy, childhood, or adolescence. With symptoms that are very different, they also have widely varying implications for the future of a child. Selective mutism, for example, although disturbing to parents and teachers, usually resolves within several months. Contrast that with separation anxiety disorder, in which long-term effects may persist for many years, or stereotypic movement disorder, in which repetitive and nonfunctional movement seriously interferes with every area of one's life. Because children are generally intolerant of those who are different, the social realities of stereotypic movement disorder can be crushing. The long-term effects can be devastating, particularly if the movements are of the self-injurious type, which can cause permanent and painful disability, even death. Fortunately, that disorder is very uncommon.

Here, we will discuss at length only separation anxiety disorder, because, of the disorders in this group, it is the one most likely to be seen, as well as to be missed as a pathology that requires treatment. It is not uncommon, with an estimated prevalence of perhaps four percent of children and young adolescents.

Unfortunately, many parents initially find the clinging and attachment behaviors endearing, not realizing the pathologic portents.

Separation Anxiety Disorder

In this disorder, the main feature is great anxiety over any type of separation from the home or from anyone to whom the child is attached. The level of anxiety over these separations is far greater than that of most children at the same developmental level. Beginning before the child is eighteen years of age, the anxiety must last at least four weeks. There is significant impairment in social, academic, or other areas of functioning. If this anxiety occurs during the course of a pervasive developmental disorder, schizophrenia, or other psychosis, the diagnosis is preempted. Adolescents who have panic disorder with agoraphobia are similarly not diagnosed with this disorder.

In children, there are a multitude of symptoms. They frequently need to know the whereabouts of their major "attachment figures" (those others, usually adults, to whom they've become most attached), and they frequently call or ask to call them by telephone. Many have reunion fantasies, even when the separation is for a relatively brief period. When away from home, they often are homesick to the point of actual physical illness. While separated, they may dwell on fears of death or injury befalling those to whom they are attached. Often they fear traveling alone and frequently fear that they will become lost and unable to rejoin their parents. School, camp, and vacations with others (other than their major attachment figures) are frightening and are avoided or actively refused. Bedtime is frequently difficult for these children, who often entreat someone to stay at their bedside until they fall asleep. Even then, they often attempt to join parents in bed. They may have frequent nightmares about their fears of losing family members through, for instance, fire, natural calamity, or violence. Quite often, these children have physical complaints when separation is imminent, such as nausea and vomiting, headaches, stomachaches, and sometimes even cardiovascular symptoms (dizziness, fainting, and palpitations). The physical complaints many times result in a medical examination that is fruitless.

For these children, most often from close-knit families, separation from significant family members frequently leads to apathy, sadness, and difficulty concentrating on important tasks (schoolwork, other responsibilities), sometimes resulting in social withdrawal. Fear and worrying about death and dying are commonly seen. When upset at the prospect of an unwanted separation (as all separations are for these children), they may become angry, striking out at those they see as causing the separation. As a group, children with this disorder are most often described as intrusive, demanding, and needing constant attention, though some are described as especially eager to please, conscientious, and compliant. Depression is often seen in these children.

This disorder can develop after a serious emotional loss or life stress (a death or serious illness in the family, loss of a pet, a geographic move). Onset can be in the preschool years, but it is most frequently seen between the start of school and the beginning of adolescence. Its course is often waxing and waning, with remission and exacerbation cycling; symptoms may abate completely or continue for years.

Important information regarding diagnosis:

• Excessive stress and anxiety in anticipating separation

• Excessive fear of losing, or harm to, major attachment figures; fear of an unusual circumstance leading to separation from these figures, such as getting lost or being kidnapped

• Reluctance or refusal to attend school or go elsewhere for fear of separation; great fear of being alone at home or elsewhere without major attachment figures

• Reluctance or refusal to go to sleep without a major attachment figure at hand or to sleep away from home

• Frequent nightmares, often about separation

• Frequent somatic complaints (stomachaches, headaches, nausea/vomiting, etc.) during separations or in anticipation of separation

• Duration of difficulties is at least four weeks; age of onset is prior to eighteen years

• The resulting disturbance results in clinically significant impairment or distress, interfering in academic, social, or other important areas of function

• Difficulties do not occur exclusively during the course of schizophrenia or other psychotic disorder, or a pervasive developmental disorder

FIVE

Major Psychiatric Illnesses

So far, we've discussed psychiatric disorders that have special significance to children and adolescents. We broadly categorized them as "developmental" in nature, because, either directly or indirectly, they all could have major roles in determining whether or not an individual grows up to be a successful, happy adult. A disorder's special significance for children arises in several ways:

- Either the disorder appears only in children or adolescents, or its onset is effectively limited to the years through adolescence

- The disorder, by definition, can be diagnosed only if its signs and symptoms begin before eighteen years of age, even though it may not achieve true significance until well into the adult years

- Although the disorder may be diagnosed at any age, its presentation in an individual's childhood or adolescence will usually presage substantial difficulties in living for the rest of that person's life; if the disorder is first acquired in adulthood, it may cause significant problems, but it will not disrupt the crucial years of development in childhood and adolescence; because normal development occurred, the affected individual will have far better tools with which to cope with problems that may arise from having that disorder

The developmental disorders we've looked at comprise only a fraction of the psychiatric diagnoses listed in the *DSM-IV*. Though significant in their contribution to the psychiatric pathology of the childhood, adolescence, and often, the entire life of the affected individual, are they the only significant psychiatric illnesses that can begin in youth?

Sadly, they are not. Other groups of psychiatric problems can be destructive to the quality of life, regardless of when they first develop. In fact, many of the most significant psychiatric illnesses often first present in adult life, so they are thought of by most people as adult psychiatric illnesses. Unfortunately for the children who develop them, they can occur at any age, sometimes with a devastation that lasts a lifetime.

Major psychiatric illnesses is the name we've chosen to refer to these so-called adult psychiatric illnesses that can affect children, usually with grave results. They all are serious mental illnesses and are most often first diagnosed in adults, but when diagnosed in childhood, they can lay waste to an otherwise successful, productive life. When they occur in a child, they usually disrupt the child's life by derailing the child's development. It's impossible to discuss in this book all the diagnoses that could potentially affect children. Our intent instead is to alert you to those other disorders that affect children very negatively with both initial presentation and long-term effects, and that you might not otherwise consider. In psychiatry, as in other branches of medicine, early detection is an important element in achieving the best outcome possible.

Schizophrenia and the Psychoses

Psychosis, regardless of type, is a disorder not well understood by most laypeople. For many people, the only contact they have had with psychosis is what they've seen in the movies or what they have read in popular works of fiction.

Although inaccurate, the notion that people who are psychotic are raving lunatics, cold-blooded serial murderers, or violent, kill-you-as-soon-as-look-at-you gang members can be close to reality. The unrealized paradox is that the diagnosis may also be accurately applied to a harmless, shy, and retiring older man who works at a socially isolated desk job as a minor clerk. His secret passion is bird-watching, and his most violent act in sixty-four years of life was once contemplating swatting at an annoying, loudly buzzing fly one hot summer's night, forty-two years earlier. He ultimately decided not to swat the fly.

Equally confusing might be the diagnosis of psychosis in a

twenty-five-year-old woman who, at five feet seven and 125 pounds, is tall and slender with long blond hair, large blue eyes, and the cheek bones of a fashion model. Although she has been described by men as "absolutely beautiful," she's had few dates and never with the same man twice. Living at home with her parents really doesn't account for her lack of social engagements. Nor does her unemployment; her father, a respected chief legal counsel for a *Fortune* 500 company, is worth millions.

Perhaps this beautiful, vivacious young woman, dressed with style and moving with grace, cools her suitor's ardor when they learn the nature of her illness.

And how could the diagnosis of psychosis be given to the delivery boy from Peterson's Grocery? He is a little small for his age and probably a little "slow," but you couldn't ask for a more dependable, pleasant, hard-working grocery delivery boy than Jerry. All afternoon he can be seen pedaling his delivery bike up and down the streets within a two-mile radius of Peterson's Grocery. Unfailingly polite, he refuses to allow women, even those larger and stronger than he, to lift or carry anything, refuses also all attempts to tip him, saying in his characteristically slow, methodical way, "No, thank you, Ma'am. Mr. Peterson pays me a living wage for my labor. It's my job, and a pleasure it's been to serve you, too. Good day!" And with that, he pedals off, returning to the store to pick up his next load of groceries.

As we said, the popular view of psychotics as being "very strange, weird, violent, and evil" is based on movies, not reality. A percentage of those with psychosis can sometimes come close to filling that bill. Yet many people with a psychosis may not be easily recognized as having an illness at all.

For example, our sixty-four-year-old clerk and bird-watcher has delusional disorder, somatic type, and has for more than twenty years. It is a type of psychosis that usually doesn't affect children, most often starting in middle or late adult life, although it can have a much earlier onset. With this disorder, the person believes that he has something wrong with his body, be it a misshapen part, foul odors, missing or nonfunctional organs, et cetera. In our example, the individual had come to believe that he had an infestation of insects growing under the skin of his arms and legs. He was understandably concerned with his "condition" and sought medical care constantly, consulting new physicians at every chance. Even though he lived in a good-sized city, he needed to call physicians' offices farther and farther from his home after he quickly ran through all the local doctors. Eventually an adult daughter who was a nurse realized what was happening with her father, moved into his home with him for a month, and took him to a psychiatrist, who started him on antipsychotic medication. It's been more than ten years since he's had the delusion, and the doses of medication he requires have actually become somewhat less.

The blond, attractive young lady suffers from schizophrenia. Suffering this particularly life-disrupting type of psychotic disorder, she actually has more difficulties than were revealed in our vignette. At nineteen years old, she was in the middle of her first year of college when she began "hearing voices." Auditory hallucinations are a common feature of schizophrenia, reported by the majority of persons with the disorder. Ultimately, the voices the woman heard resolved to one male voice. The voice frequently taunted her, and eventually her psychiatrist, through her reports of the content of the voice's speech, was able to delineate the details of a complex delusional system the young woman had developed.

By the time the psychiatrist was initially contacted, this young woman's father had withdrawn her from the university and had moved her home. Hoping that what was happening to her was only a temporary aberration, her parents attempted to take care of her on their own. Though they had no reason to believe she used psychedelic drugs, they allowed themselves to believe that perhaps she had taken or been "slipped" some LSD, resulting in her condition. During the next two months, however, they were forced by the intensity of her obvious delusions to acknowledge that whatever the mechanism, their daughter was very seriously ill.

The male voice she began hearing soon became identified to her as Phillipus, a man from the planet Venus. She confided to her psychiatrist that "Phillipus" was not actually his name, but that he'd told her that she could never pronounce his Venusian name—"Phillipus" was the closest sound to his actual name that he thought an English-speaking person could pronounce. He was the equivalent on Venus of a two-star general on Earth, he'd told her, and was in charge of interplanetary espionage. Using Venusian technology, he'd spied her one day with his imaging equipment and noticed how the male students had attended to her at the university. Because she was so attractive to human males and because most heads of state on Earth were male, he thought she might be useful to him as an agent—as a spy.

The details of the rest of her hallucinations and delusions are not important here. What is important to know is that when she first spoke to her psychiatrist, she completely believed that she was in daily contact with "Phillipus" and that he had arranged the implantation in her head of a miniature transmitter/receiver both to transmit her thoughts to him and to receive his thoughts in her mind. Although her medications help reduce the effect of her schizophrenia to more moderate levels, she's currently too ill for her hallucinations and delusions to completely resolve. Hopefully, over time, her illness will remit sufficiently for her medications to free her from them.

And Jerry, the delivery boy? He, too, is psychotic. His is a type of psychosis that literally defies specific diagnosis; it's called psychotic disorder, not otherwise specified (NOS). In this type of psychosis, the patient presents clearly psychotic symptoms (for instance, hallucinations, delusions, very disorganized behavior or speech, et cetera). Even though the symptoms may be obviously psychotic, there may be inadequate information to fill the criteria for any specific psychotic disorder, hence, psychotic disorder, NOS.

Jerry's birth was a breech presentation. His already difficult delivery was complicated by the umbilical cord's being wrapped around his throat. His development seemed relatively normal in the perinatal period after a somewhat lowered Apgar (a rating of a newborn's apparent health) at birth, but by the sixth month of life, it was clear to all that Jerry had sustained some permanent brain damage. Left with a small but clinically significant intellectual deficit (IQ tested at 65), Jerry was eventually diagnosed with mild mental retardation. His physical development also appeared to have been affected: Jerry was always the shortest male in his age group through school. A slow but hard worker, Jerry continued in school in special education. Though it was not reported when it first occurred (apparently at age seven) by the time Jerry was ten, he could contain himself no longer. He told his parents of the voices he heard. Though he never reported other psychotic symptoms or evidenced any psychotic signs, the child and adolescent psychiatrist his parents consulted diagnosed Jerry as having psychotic disorder, NOS.

A small but important dose of antipsychotic medication, also known as a neuroleptic, quieted the voices almost to silence. Except for occasional exacerbations—most likely occasioned by overwhelming life stress, such as when his favorite aunt, Linda, was hospitalized for a week with congestive heart failure—Jerry plugged along, slowly but surely winning everyone's affection with his mild temper, ready smile, and hard work.

Even though the last three individuals discussed are, in fact, good examples of people with psychosis, there really are individuals whose psychotic illness enables them to perform acts seen by others as depraved, who feel no guilt for those acts, or who actually enjoy doing what others see as "evil works." If they all have the same illness, why is it that some are gentle and harmless, whereas others are able to perform unspeakable acts?

To learn the answer, one must first understand, at least in basic terms, what psychosis really is. Various definitions have been used through the years, ranging from a restrictive definition that says psychosis is limited to those conditions that produce delusions or hallucinations as their primary features, to variations on this theme, including whether or not the individual has insight and can understand the hallucinations as being pathological.

Schizophrenia and other psychotic disorders focus on different aspects of what we consider psychosis, whether it's prominent hallucinations, delusions, or disorganized speech or behavior. Unrecognized and untreated, psychotic disorders may imply for an individual a hellish existence or only a reputation for being "a little strange, but harmless." The wide range of effects from psychosis results from the differences in seriousness from disorder to disorder. Although popular perceptions of these disorders are often exaggerated, there are those people so deranged that protection of themselves and others requires their hospitalization.

There is much evidence to suggest psychotic disorders may be in part linked to genetic factors. Various types of psychosis tend to cluster within a family. Often, where a number of people in a family share some psychotic disturbances, their behavior and thought process may be considered normal within that family.

Sometimes the cause of psychosis is not genetically related, but rather is a physiological consequence of a general medical condition (such as uncontrolled diabetes, high fever, thyroid disorder, et cetera). Most frequently, these brief psychoses resolve completely as the medical condition causing them is treated effectively. A second major cause of psychosis unrelated to inheritance is the use or abuse of various substances. For example, serious abuse of cocaine or amphetamines can cause a short-term psychosis. Authorities in large cities often pick up one or two heavy cocaine abusers a night suffering from terrifying paranoid delusions and hallucinations.

In children generally (and even more so in younger children), it can be difficult to become alerted to the presence of a psychotic disorder, because a number of the signs of psychosis could be seen as normal childhood behaviors. In fact, childlike behaviors in adults are what makes it difficult to be with a psychotic adult for long without realizing that something is wrong.

Children, however, are "allowed" to have mythical friends, to "see" them where adults cannot, to "hear" them when adults cannot, and to hold conversations with them. What parent would immediately think that their child was experiencing visual and auditory hallucinations if she pretended to have an imaginary friend? When a young boy watches the movie *E.T.* and for days after behaves like the character, E.T., we think it's cute. We do not think him delusional or psychotic. If he were, in fact, psychotic, it might take days—maybe even a week—before we realized that he wasn't just a child with a fanciful imagination.

Ideas of reference—the term for a psychotic individual's belief that information coming over the radio or television, or even printed in a newspaper, is specifically directed to him—is fairly easy to detect in an adult. Because children are still much more concrete in their understanding of the world than are adults, they may genuinely believe that the radio or TV is speaking directly to them without being thought of as psychotic (even though they could be). Our point here is that children and sometimes even adolescents may manifest signs and symptoms of psychosis that initially go unrecognized by the adults who love and care for them. Because children are allowed and even expected to use their imaginations in play, none of the major symptoms of psychosis (hallucinations, delusions, disorganized speech, disorganized behavior) in a young child would cause the immediate concern that they would in an adult. Quite often, the first time a parent realizes that something is wrong is when the child, acting on delusional beliefs or following the prompting of hallucinatory voices, acts in such a bizarre way that it's impossible to ignore.

Rather than wait for that inescapable incident, take note of the following symptoms and consult a child mental health provider to discuss their meaning if you detect them:

- What was once a fantasy thought has become a rigid, fixed belief to your child—one he holds as if it were real

- When your child pretends to be listening to an invisible friend, you realize that they are not pretending

- Strange or unusual beliefs that were once readily identified as make-believe (you knew your child didn't actually believe they were real) now seem real to the child

Modern psychiatry has learned much; the treatment of mildly psychotic patients today is almost uniformly administered on an outpatient basis. Although seriously ill psychotics are likely to be hospitalized for a significant portion of their lives, conditions have improved tremendously. Medications that weren't dreamed of at the turn of the century have long since freed many from their personal demons and improved the quality of life for countless others. Advances in brain imaging, neurochemistry, and an ever-increasing appreciation of neurophysiology have led us away from punitive, ineffective treatments. Today, treatments for psychosis are constantly being refined in pharmacological company laboratories; more effective treatments are being developed today for use tomorrow. The future holds the promise of the time when psychosis will be as readily curable as polio is readily preventable today.

Mood Disorders

Although common sense argues that many psychiatric disorders affect the individual's mood, the term *mood disorders* has a specific meaning in psychiatry. In *DSM-IV*, the term refers to two families of disorders: depressive disorders and bipolar disorders. Much psychiatric and psychological research in recent years has been performed in these areas due to the large numbers of people who suffer from these disorders and the economic impact they have on our nation. Problems such as physical illness and accidents take a larger toll on people with depressive disorders than on otherwise healthy people. That is, depressed people miss more school or work and have more accidents involving injury than do those who are not depressed. People with bipolar disorder, too, have higher rates of physical illness and accidents than in the general population. Both groups of disorders can have effects that range from relatively harmless to life-shattering. Unfortunately, children are immune to neither.

Depressive Disorders

The depressive disorders consist of three diagnoses: major depressive disorder, dysthymic disorder, and depressive disorder not otherwise specified (NOS). As most people realize, depressive symptoms can range from being mildly "blue" to the depths of depression accompanied by feelings of helplessness and hopelessness encountered with severe depression. Some people believe that depression is a disorder reserved for lonely or sick older people. There is a bit of truth there, in that older people, and especially older people who have chronic or serious illness and who are alone, frequently have a depressive disorder. Sad as that might be, however, the pediatric and adolescent populations can also suffer crippling major depression.

Most of us use our commonsense understanding of the term *depression* when we consider a friend or acquaintance to be depressed. Because all of us have been sad, unhappy, down in the dumps, or feeling blue, we can relate to others who feel similarly. We can even make comments such as "Bill seems a little down today" or "Sue acts really sad" or "I think Mr. Johnson is really depressed; he hasn't eaten lunch all week, and he looks like he hasn't slept in a month!" Usually, our observations are more accurate than we realize.

Depression in adults usually presents signs that almost anyone can recognize, though even in adults we sometimes miss the signs that would tell us someone is clinically depressed. Depression in children, however, may present itself in ways that we don't classically associate with depression. As a result, we can fail to recognize certain behaviors and attitudes as stemming from depressive illness. This can be an important problem, because untreated depression can cause serious difficulties with school, behavior, and personal relationships. Recognizing and obtaining effective treatment for depression are just as important for children as they are for adults. Some authorities suggest that they may be even more important in the case of a child, because the developmental years have such a profound effect on the rest of an individual's life. If a child is seriously depressed during that time and goes untreated, how much will his overall development suffer as a result? And how much of an effect will that have on his success later in life?

Recognizing that your child is depressed is just as important as knowing she has a major physical illness. Certain signs of depression are fairly universal across age groups; we'll discuss those first. Many people who are experiencing depression also show signs of appetite change, along with other so-called *vegetative signs*. Whereas adults who are depressed may either eat a great deal more, a great deal less, or almost stop eating altogether, children generally respond to depression by having less appetite. Even favorite meals and desserts can lose their appeal. Many times parents correctly interpret their child's lack of appetite by recognizing other factors affecting her on a one-time basis, such as gastrointestinal upset. Be aware that many causes for decreased appetite can occur intermittently. If you notice that your child is not eating well for a long period of time (more than a week), it is a good idea to have a little chat with her to determine if there is another physical reason for the loss of appetite or if it's related to anticipation or worry about a specific event (a big test next Monday, a school dance, et cetera). If there seems to be no physiological cause for loss of appetite and no acute event took place a day or two before or is anticipated in the next week or so, investigate further.

Sleep habits are also frequently affected by depression. As in adults, children may show a need for increased sleep or an increased difficulty in falling or staying asleep. Particularly in young children, increasing incidence of nightmares can tip you off to a problem with depression and worry.

Anhedonia—the loss of pleasure from, or interest in, favored activities—often signals possible problems with depression. For example, if your fourteen-year-old son would usually rather drive a go-cart than eat, but an offer to take him to the local go-cart track is met with a bored look and a sighed, "No, thanks, Dad, I just don't feel like it today," it doesn't necessarily mean your son is depressed. But you might want to check with other family members to see if they have noticed anything unusual about him. A private chat may also be in order.

Psychomotor behaviors such as fidgeting and other minor movements as well as manner and rate of speech can tell you a lot about how your child is feeling. When your child is depressed or anxious, her psychomotor activity may increase; conversely, her manner of speech may become more laconic, and you may hear many more one- or two-word replies to questions than usual—even in teenagers. You may also notice that the rate of speech has slowed and the tone is flatter, less expressive. A depressed child may sometimes appear less animated than usual. A child who fidgets more than usual and sits around the house more, sighing and looking blue, is giving you a good reason to suggest taking a walk together and touching base; something's on her mind.

Most children and teenagers have enormous reserves of energy and are normally active. A child or teenager who reports feeling low energy and is not interested in his normal activities or who seems too tired to participate may be showing signs of depression. If your child appears to be or complains of being tired all the time, and small amounts of exertion result in sustained fatigue, consider the possibility of depression. It's also important to consider that the child's fatigue or lack of energy may be caused by a physical illness, as well. If with these complaints he also tells you he feels ill, has nausea or vomiting, or other signs of flu or similar ailments, a doctor visit is in order. Keep in mind that depression or other emotional upset can also cause physical complaints, particularly in children.

In fact, physical complaints such as headaches, stomachaches, nausea, and other flulike symptoms are often associated with depression—especially when reported with greater frequency than usual. If an otherwise healthy child or teenager suddenly has multiple, nonspecific physical complaints, a screening by the child's pediatrician is a good idea. Not only can the doctor screen for serious illness, she often is able to elicit information from a child that he might be reluctant to tell a parent.

Feelings of worthlessness and guilt, as well as feelings of low self-esteem, often accompany depressed mood. These feelings may signal a more serious depression. A child who displays any of the other signs mentioned earlier, who cries easily and more frequently than usual, and who feels worthless or guilty may be seriously depressed. Although no one wants to be an alarmist, we believe that multiple, serious signs of depression, whether in a five-year-old or a fifteen-year-old, need attention immediately.

A major complication in evaluating a child for depression is that most parents who recognize the obvious signs may never recognize that there are other signs, some subtle, some not so subtle, that can indicate a serious depression. A child who suddenly and uncharacteristically begins to fight with siblings or who "talks back" and is disrespectful in school, at home, or with friends may be displaying depression atypically. Children who have been model citizens who start acting out in school, frequently getting into trouble, or who start an inexplainable period of bad behavior (for a young child) or so-called delinquent behavior—staying out past curfew, breaking windows, painting slogans on walls, shoplifting, slashing tires, engaging in assaultive behavior—may be acting out their frustration and anger. This acting out is often a sign of depression.

Likewise, poor academic performance in a child who usually does well in school or a noticeable decline in effort may be the only indication you have that a child is depressed. Difficulty thinking or concentrating effectively may be another sign of depression. Clearly, these signs need to be followed up with a mental health professional.

Clinically significant depression may be of the major depression type, where the symptoms are usually more severe and have been ongoing for a longer time, or it may be of a dysthymic type, which is low grade, but lasts for a long time. Dysthymia, though not as dangerous or disruptive as major depression, still represents a major block to your child's happiness and overall success in life—it drains much of his intellectual and emotional energy. The dysthymic child deserves treatment every bit as much as the child with major depression.

Bipolar Disorder

Bipolar disorder is the current name for what was once called manic-depression. Today, this disorder is considered to have two types, I and II; the distinguishing factor relates to the severity of the manic phase. In our discussion, we'll consider the two types equivalent for our purpose.

This disorder can lead to lifelong difficulties of major proportion or allow a mostly productive, effective life. Several factors influence which path is followed. The first factor is genetic. The degree to which the disorder has the potential to be treated effectively is largely determined by how pervasive the disorder is in a specific individual. This is mainly established by the genetic component of the disorder. A second factor is the family support the child receives. If the family of that child is supportive, understanding, and willing to help the child help himself by participating as needed in the therapeutic program, the long-term prognosis may well be improved.

Another important factor that may lessen the overall effect the disorder has on the child's life is the earliest possible detection and evaluation of the bipolar disorder. Many parents of a child with bipolar disorder are unable (or unwilling) to face the implications of their child's having a serious psychiatric illness. A more effective way to deal with those implications, of course, is to learn what one can about the disorder, then do what one must to help the child continue to develop as completely as she can.

Other disorders or problems sometimes associated with bipolar disorder include school problems, social difficulties, attention deficit hyperactivity disorder, panic disorder, bulimia, anorexia nervosa, social phobia, and substance abuse. Of course, not all of these problems and disorders occur in everyone with bipolar disorder, nor will any one individual with bipolar disorder necessarily have any of these other problems.

Treatment of bipolar disorder has improved over time, as it has with most psychiatric illnesses; breakthroughs expected soon after the turn of the century promise to increase the help we can offer to those with this disorder. Current treatment can include psychotherapy, but most often is medication-based. Medication used for bipolar disorder includes representatives from several chemical classes. The most commonly used medications are those called "mood stabilizers," and they are sometimes used in other disorders where the potential for manic behavior is high.

People with bipolar disorder may experience a widely diverse number of episodes, classified as major depressive episodes, manic episodes, or hypomanic episodes. (Major depressive episodes are associated with both bipolar I and bipolar II disorder; hypomania, which is a somewhat less exuberant type of mania, is associated with bipolar II disorder; mania, with bipolar I disorder.) Frequency of episodes and total lifetime episodes also vary greatly. Medication doesn't offer complete protection against either depressive or manic episodes, but it seems today to be the most effective thing that can be done to prevent future episodes.

Unfortunately, both types have about the same number of completed suicides—ten to fifteen percent. Although there is some difference in the numbers between bipolar I and II, most people with either return to a fully functional state between episodes. However, intervals between episodes decrease as one ages. Both types are associated with psychotic features, though not all who have bipolar disorder will ever display psychosis. After an episode in which psychotic features are noted, however, the likelihood of psychosis being related to future episodes increases.

Manic episodes represent a distinct period during which the individual expresses an abnormal and persistent moJod that's elevated, expansive, or irritable. For a person to qualify for the diagnosis, this altered mood must last for at least a week; less is acceptable if the person is hospitalized for treatment. Some of the other possible symptoms include:

• Greatly inflated self-esteem or grandiosity

• Decreased need for sleep

• Pressured, often rapid, speech

• Flight of ideas, wherein the individual's thoughts and speech race from topic to topic

• Greatly increased distractibility, with otherwise irrelevant stimuli capturing his attention

In mania, the individual may become very goal oriented and directed, though after the mania abates, she may see that the focus of her activity was not a valuable goal at all. The last symptom is one that most people have seen in the movies—the attention to pleasurable activities, completely without concern for the consequences: the spending of cash or credit on purchases that the person wouldn't consider in a normal state; unwise business dealings; sexual activity that would normally be avoided, such as promiscuity, et cetera.

Many people with bipolar disorder are successful and productive when not in a manic state, recovering to normal between episodes. So they are often ashamed and embarrassed by their unrestrained behavior while manic. Aside from the risks of financial ruin, infection with sexually transmitted diseases, and great embarrassment, people in a manic state risk physical injury when pursuing high-risk, exciting pastimes; even driving an automobile can be dangerous, because a manic at the wheel probably will not drive in her normal, conservative manner. Very sadly, many people in a manic episode have been injured or killed while pursuing a goal. A large number of others have been arrested, convicted, and imprisoned for crimes they committed while in a manic state. An irritable manic is at much increased risk for violent behavior directed toward family members, friends, even total strangers.

Even though bipolar disorder is not as common in children as it is in adults, it is included here because it can be seen in children. It is almost never recognized because of a depressive episode, but rather for the manic episode. Prompt diagnosis is unlikely, since the incidence in children is much lower than that in adults. Occasionally children in a manic state are mistakenly diagnosed as ADHD, but that error is generally corrected shortly, since children with bipolar disorder not in a manic state do not resemble hyperactive children at all, unless the child has ADHD as well as bipolar disorder. Typically, a child with ADHD, if hyperactive, is hyperactive fairly consistently.

Anxiety Disorders

Earlier in the book we discussed anxiety difficulties common (though not exclusively) in children. Here, we will look at several of the disorders identified only as anxiety disorders. Although most people think of the disorders included under this heading as fairly exclusive to adults, children also fall prey to them.

Anxiety disorders can be frightening and destabilizing. Adults who have these disorders are sometimes incapacitated by the emotional distress the symptoms cause. Small wonder, then, that children also can have great difficulty with them!

A common thread is woven through the anxiety disorders; in virtually every situation in which any of these disorders is experienced, there are usually somatic symptoms that reflect the intensity of the anxiety. Most are distinctly unpleasant; those people who anticipate them will often go to great lengths to avoid experiencing them. They can include:

- A pounding or rapidly beating heart

- Sweating, trembling, or shaking

- Shortness of breath or a smothering sensation

- Choking

- Chest pain

- Nausea or abdominal discomfort

- Dizziness, lightheadedness, or fainting

- Fear that one is "going crazy" or losing control

- Fear of dying

- Tingling or numbness, usually in the limbs

- Hot flashes or chills

Certainly, not all symptoms listed occur simultaneously, but any one or two would be sufficient to dismay almost anyone.

The anxiety disorders are a complex series of disorders with many variations on a theme. The theme is that of worry and anxiety concerning an experience that evokes great fear and concern or a future event that one fears will happen in a way that will cause embarrassment or discomfort, emotionally or physically. The individual may not always be consciously aware of the source of the anxiety. Dealing with the spectrum of anxiety disorders takes a considerable amount of time and energy from those who suffer with them, often leaving far less of either than necessary to be truly effective in their lives. For those with social phobia, specific phobia, or panic disorder with or without agoraphobia, much of their energy and concern is spent avoiding those situations or things that produce their anxiety. Quite a few people have been unable to go to work or school or to maintain social relationships because of fears and anxieties evoked by traveling from home, flying or driving, working or living in certain environments, et cetera.

Consider, then, how the stress and anxiety—and the physical symptoms that can accompany them—would affect a young child, a seventh grader, a high school senior. Although it's true that in some ways our children may have it better than we did at their age, we also didn't have many of the pressures that they experience. The world has changed. Children and adolescents also lack the protection given to us by our experience in life and the world. Anxiety disorders rob everyone who has them of pieces of their lives, but children are especially vulnerable.

Let's survey some of the most significant anxiety disorders:

Panic attacks are discrete periods during which the individual experiences a sudden sense of impending doom with apprehension and fear. Many of the symptoms we discussed at the beginning of the chapter accompany this sense, such as a pounding heart, choking, and shortness of breath. *Agoraphobia* is anxiety about going places where escape might be either difficult or embarrassing or where help for panic attacks might not be available should a person have one. Panic disorder may occur with or without accompanying agoraphobia.

Specific phobias are characterized by significant anxiety caused by exposure to feared objects or situations such as water, high places, or animals. Avoidance of the feared object or situation often becomes a debilitating obsession.

Social phobias also often lead to the formation of avoidance. Fears and anxiety are caused by a specific type of social or performance situation. The child who is afraid to read aloud in class because he fears being embarrassed by mispronouncing a word and the older child who fears giving an oral report in front of the class because he feels others will see his hands shaking may both have a social phobia.

Anxiety can also be a physiological result of a general medical condition or of posttraumatic stress disorder (PTSD), first identified in war veterans and now recognized in children, especially those who've been physically or sexually abused or who've been in a serious accident or natural disaster. This disorder is discussed in more detail in chapter seven.

Obsessive-Compulsive Disorder (OCD) is somewhat different from the others in the anxiety group. It's characterized by obsessions that cause great anxiety and compulsions that, when acted out, relieve the anxiety. Although OCD is a significant diagnosis by itself, it is frequently associated with many other disorders. It is often seen with attention deficit hyperactivity disorder as a comorbid (simultaneous) condition; in a similar fashion, it is also associated with Tourette's disorder and the other tic disorders, autistic disorder, Asperger's disorder, and a number of other psychiatric illnesses.

OCD can be very problematic. For reasons we don't yet understand, a particular thought or idea becomes very important to the person with OCD. Over time, he thinks about it more and more. The thought is disturbing to him; it is intrusive and inappropriate and causes him anxiety that he is unable to relieve. Compulsions are repetitive behaviors that are performed in the hope of reducing the anxiety produced by the obsession. The individual is driven to perform the compulsion. For a short while after, relief from the anxiety is obtained, and the cycle is reset. A frequently given example is that of a child or adult who is obsessed with a concern about germs. Every time he touches a doorknob or other objects or shakes hands (if he even will)—after doing almost everything one does with hands—he feels compelled to wash his hands to cleanse them of dangerous germs.

Of course, human skin was not designed to be washed with caustic soaps fifty times a day. As he continues washing, he eventually can develop open sores. Even with that pain, if he continues to harbor the obsession, he'll still wash his hands at the first thought of contamination.

In children, OCD may be associated with wish fulfillment thoughts—like that of a young boy approaching puberty who had never thought of climbing into a garbage Dumpster and rummaging until he drove past one on his bike one day. "It was like there was, you know, maybe a treasure in there! Maybe a computer . . . maybe a dirt bike! I got really excited, you know? Like I *had* to check it out! I didn't know, but I did know I had to get in there and look!" Later in the conversation he was asked what he thought and felt as he was trying to resist the urge to climb into the Dumpster. "Well, I did think, 'I'm not supposed to go near those,' but the feeling . . . the excitement . . . of the thought of the good stuff that might be in there . . . it took over, you know? . . . the urge to look was very strong . . . I had to do it!" How did he feel after he'd looked? "Well, I didn't find much that was any good, but I kinda relaxed, like I wasn't so . . . so wired, ya know? On other days I'd ride past it, but I didn't think of it. Then I'd ride past it again, and I'd know I had to look that day . . . I'd get wired, my brain felt weird, ya know?"

This youngster was punished each time his parents found that he'd climbed into one of the Dumpsters—but he continued until his mother took him to see a child psychiatrist. His mother, Kathy, explains: "We'd had trouble keeping Kevin out of the Dumpsters. Neither his father nor I could believe that he'd even think of going into the filthy things! But he did, and pretty frequently. We grounded him, took away privileges . . . but nothing ever helped. One of my friends had taken her son to see this psychiatrist for ADHD, and was very pleased . . . so we went to see him. He asked a lot of questions about Kevin's life up until then . . . and I realized that he'd been doing some things he'd been told not to for about two years. Kevin's no angel, but he'd been a pretty obedient kid, so we just didn't understand this behavior." One afternoon while getting a lecture from his mom about going into the Dumpsters again, Kevin told her how he'd felt as he looked at the Dumpsters. Kathy continues, "So I thought that that sounded pretty strange. His father and I talked about it that night. We agreed Kevin needed to see a child psychiatrist."

The doctor had determined that Kevin was depressed and would start him, with Kathy's permission, on a small dose of a new type of antidepressant that would help with his depression and with what the doctor believed was OCD.

"In less than a week," Kathy said, "Kevin really did seem to lighten up, to feel better, and he told me he didn't feel like going into the Dumpsters again. They were really dirty and terrible smelling, and he'd never found a treasure anyway!"

It's very important to note that Kevin—usually a good child—was being punished for willfully disobeying. His behavior—which he had no control over—was initially labeled as defiant and oppositional. Yet his OCD made it effectively impossible not to go into the Dumpsters. No one but Kevin even knew of his struggle, and for a while, he was seen as a "bad" child.

Not all obsessive-compulsive behavior is exactly like this.

This is a good example, though, because it illustrates the disorder well. The excitement that Kevin had felt looking at the Dumpster overpowered his desire to be obedient.

In young people especially, OCD can be an important component of a multifactorial—many-faceted—behavioral problem. In Kevin's case, it became clear that he had a number of obsessions involving behaviors that had been forbidden. They all resolved with the use of the antidepressant. Sometimes, though, therapy is needed to break the OCD cycle; medication is not enough. In an older child or adolescent, both cognitive and behavioral therapy might prove very helpful (see chapter ten).

Eating Disorders

Today's media discuss eating disorders on an almost daily basis. Unfortunately, some segments of the media *promote* eating disorders as well by publicizing ridiculous and unsafe diets. Yet the American preoccupation with weight and appearance is all too real. So, too, are the deaths and serious illnesses caused by anorexia nervosa and bulimia nervosa.

Strongly related in outcome, anorexia and bulimia focus on a fear of gaining weight; they differ in their approach to the "problem." In anorexia nervosa, the central feature is that the individual refuses to maintain a normal body and is intensely afraid of gaining weight. She also has a disturbed body image, seeing herself as "fat," regardless of what the tape measure or scale indicates. Bulimia nervosa addresses the "problem" somewhat differently: Bulimics routinely binge eat, then use inappropriate compensating methods, such as purging (self-induced vomiting) and often the chronic use of laxatives and diuretics.

A common misconception is that these two dangerous disorders occur only in late adolescence and early adulthood. Yet, every day medical centers around the country report the deaths of young people who died after unsuccessfully battling anorexia or bulimia.

In America, these disorders primarily affect females; the ratio is reported as approximately nine or ten to one, female to male. Although boys and young men are also concerned about appearance, occupational success, and being sexually attractive, they learn that they can achieve acceptance by being productive, working hard, and so forth. Some people working in the eating disorders field believe that anorexia and bulimia are the logical result of sexism. They feel that many young women, despite the enormous social and economic advances women have made in recent decades, still become convinced that the only way they'll ever achieve financial and social security is by finding and marrying the right man. Even that famous, slender, long-legged doll of our childhood, Barbie, hasn't escaped censure and blame: It's been estimated that the average American girl has approximately eight of these popular dolls. As you'll remember, this doll has an exaggerated figure, with a waist tiny in relation to her hips. Her critics maintain that she is at least partially responsible for the obsession that many young American women have with being extremely slender. Further, recent examinations of children's attitudes showed that children overwhelmingly associated physical appearance with personality traits. Shown a picture of an attractive woman, children invariably responded that she was "nice," "friendly," and that "everybody likes her."

Regardless of the motivation for the fear of fat and the obsession with being slender, increasing numbers of American women are damaging their physical and mental health by engaging in incredibly restrictive diets and excessive exercise. This pattern, characteristic of anorexia, results in an enormous amount of psychic pain, physical illness, and, occasionally, death. (Singer Karen Carpenter is reported to have died of a heart ailment attributed to anorexia.) Similar findings are reported for bulimia. Usually within the normal weight range (some are slightly above or below ideal body weight), these women routinely restrict their caloric intake and use "diet" foods between binges.

Though there are differences between anorexia and bulimia, both are dangerous disorders that reflect serious pathology regarding one's self-image and how one determines self-worth. When someone with anorexia or bulimia looks in the mirror, instead of seeing herself as others do (for the most part, to be a little underweight, rather than overweight) they see themselves as "fat." Sufferers of both disorders may be overheard to say things like, "I'm just too fat," "I'm ugly," "I'd be okay if only I had thinner (legs, thighs, hips)," "I never do anything right," or "I'm a failure." These people risk serious illness and death to achieve the acceptance of others. Because acceptance of self is never really achieved, they never feel accepted by others and will continue to focus inappropriately on food and eating.

Adolescent girls especially are likely to lie about laxative use or purging. If these teenagers are seriously underweight, they may constantly complain about being cold, since they've lost much of their insulating layer of fat. They may complain of being dizzy or lightheaded, of feeling faint, or of tingling in the hands, feet, or face. Malnutrition, dehydration, and hormonal imbalances may cause frequent or constant headaches, brittle hair, dry skin, bruising, and bleeding gums. If they are purging frequently (bulimia), there may be a loss of tooth enamel from the effects of acid in the mouth. They may exercise for hours at a time. At mealtimes, they may excuse themselves, claiming lack of hunger or that they don't feel well. If forced to eat with the family, they may do little more than move things around on their plates, actually eating very little.

With both disorders, effective and immediate therapy is necessary. If a parent notices any of these signs of eating disorders on a regular or continuous basis, evaluation by an eating disorder specialist is strongly recommended. Almost without exception, initial evaluation and treatment should be in an inpatient setting, with careful follow-up in the postdischarge period. An eating disorder can put a child's immediate and future health—both mental and physical—at risk. The sooner the pattern is interrupted, the better.

Substance Abuse

On every television station in the country, it seems, there are daily public service announcements produced by federal and state governments in which movie stars, sports figures, and others exhort our youth not to start using drugs and alcohol or to stop using them immediately. Yet even with all this, more and more American youth choose to "turn on, toke up, and get high." Although massive antidrug campaigns have slowed down the involvement of some segments of our youth, other segments have continued to use and abuse drugs and alcohol. Some have actually increased their use and abuse.

There are no simple solutions to the problem of drug abuse in this country; the flow of illegal drugs into this country seems unabated, despite all efforts. Targeting messages to those considered most vulnerable to substance abuse seems to have failed. Rather than address those larger concerns, we focus here on the importance of the parents' ability to recognize substance abuse in their children and to give their children the help they need.

Many books have been written on substance abuse, especially substance abuse among adolescents. Some take one point of view, some take another. Yet they all agree on one thing: Prevention is far more valuable than treatment, but if prevention fails, the sooner treatment starts, the greater the likelihood of success.

Prevention

Children adopt many of the attitudes and behaviors of their parents. When we're young and living at home, we learn by example, modeling ourselves after our same-gender parent. So when we speak of prevention of any behavior in our children, we need to be aware that their first lesson in what they'll accept as appropriate behavior comes from *our* behavior. When the grandfather counseled his grandson not to drink alcohol, the grandson objected, "But Grandfather! You drink alcohol!" Grandfather replied quickly, "That's true. But you must do as I say, not as I do." Perhaps that might work in children's stories, but it doesn't in real life. Your behavior is one of the most powerful ways you communicate with your children.

Telling your children not to smoke as you light up your thirtieth cigarette of the day is probably not the most effective message you'll give that day. As your son and daughter help you clean up the mess in the family room the morning after an adult party, with empty beer bottles, half-empty whiskey decanters, and overflowing ashtrays, your appeal to their better judgment as you tell them not to drink will seem hollow and hypocritical. To be effective in helping your children avoid substance abuse, you must first examine your own beliefs and behaviors and make some basic decisions about your true feelings on the subject. Communicating with your children one way with words and a different way with behavior will not confuse them for long.

Perhaps you've always been a responsible role model. You've done everything you could to dissuade your children from the use of drugs and alcohol. Should you remain concerned about what they might do anyway? In a word, yes.

Continue to talk to your children about your feelings concerning substance abuse and about your wish that, regardless of the pressure they feel from peers to use these substances, they will refrain. Encourage them to come to you to discuss concerns, fears, and difficulties they may be experiencing. Remember, though, that if you encourage their confidence in you, and you promise to take no punitive action based on what they say, you must hold up your end of the bargain. Coming from a position of trust, giving your children your trust, and encouraging them to talk with you may go a long way in preventing many problems as they grow up.

When Should I Become Concerned?

Despite your hard efforts, your trust, and your love, it's still possible that your child may choose to use drugs and alcohol. Although you'll probably feel disappointed and concerned if this happens, "losing your cool" might just make things worse.

Instead of making your child's life miserable by constantly asking about her use or nonuse of drugs, be aware of how she behaves and what seems to be going on in her life. As you monitor her attitudes and behavior, be especially vigilant for:

- A previously good student who starts to do poorly in all his subjects at school

- A teen with a better driving record than yours who starts to have "fender benders"

- A previously talkative and outgoing youth who no longer shares with you any details of her life, especially about her whereabouts when not at home. (Keep in mind that as adolescents get older, being more private is natural—but if she cuts you off totally, it should concern you)

- Excessive sniffling or coughing

- Hair and clothing that smells like smoke

- Vagueness and even evasiveness when your teenager is asked about friends and outside activities, even considering his increased need for privacy

- A neat child who becomes increasingly messy

- A "clotheshorse" who loses interest in her appearance

- Drug paraphernalia: rolling papers, pipes, decongestant bottles, eyedrops

- Incense, other scents used to "cover up"

- Drugs or signs of drugs: pills, white powder, plant leaves or seeds in ashtrays or pockets, hypodermic needles

- Drug slogans on clothes, magazines about drugs

- A child who gets angry when you discuss drug use

- A previously sharp adolescent who has memory lapses or difficulty in concentrating

- Dilated or "pinpoint" pupils

- Obvious lying or evidence of stealing

- Increased irritability or unwillingness to cooperate

- Lower levels of energy, self-discipline, motivation, self-esteem

If your child displays more than two or three of the traits or circumstances just listed, concern is warranted. With more than five, consider having your child meet with a mental health professional who specializes in adolescent substance abuse. Substance abuse is a frightening topic for a parent to consider. If your child is abusing drugs or alcohol, your greatest need is for immediate help for your child—and for you.

You will need to be at your best and strongest to be able to be there for your child as he needs you, but you also will need to be strong enough to resist him when he attempts to manipulate you to avoid immediate therapy. Violence and loud, angry arguments won't help; if they did, few children would abuse. Don't push your child away before you can try to help. Save your initial shock or anger for a therapist's office, where you can also learn how best to help and guide your child.

If your child is abusing substances, prepare yourself for her attempts to dissuade you, to get you to believe no problem exists. The substance and the problem your child may have developed with it are stronger than her good logic and common sense. Don't allow them to be stronger than yours. Consult the most experienced professional you can locate about your concerns before you broach the subject with your child.

You owe your child your love and concern. You also owe her the best you can do to help her. Don't, however, enable her. Dealing effectively with her problem will be hard work. Don't attempt to make it easier; you might destroy the effectiveness of her growth. You help your child best by supporting a well-trained therapist, not your child's efforts to "escape."

Making Sense of Your Child's Problems in School

School should be one of the most fun and rewarding experiences in any child's life. In a perfect world, it would be. In our far-from-perfect world, however, going to school more often presents new ways and places to get into trouble. Even so, school gives parents an incredible opportunity to learn more about their children.

By maintaining close communication with an interested and caring faculty, parents can often learn how effectively their child relates to other children and authority figures and can gain insight to other areas of importance. Parents can learn, for example, how their child seems to learn best (through hearing, seeing, or hands-on experience) and work that style of learning into more casual but still important teaching at home about many important topics. Finding out what's most effective for a child in learning new material can also help parents help their child to gain more from the other, less-used modes of learning. Parents will also benefit from learning about their child's style of relating to others. If the child is positive, enthusiastic, and respectful of others—both peers and supervising adults—parents can reinforce those traits. If it's the opposite, parents can intervene and help the child learn more effective styles of relating, without causing the child to feel bad or wrong about the old ways. If there are serious problems with the child's performance in school, with his apparent ability to learn, or with his manner of relating to authority figures or peers, involved parents will learn sooner and be in a better position to intervene or seek professional help.

Poor school performance can be directly related to strife in the home, but poor school performance can also be related to other factors. Of course, poor academic performance, relationship difficulties, and behavior problems can also be related to emotional or psychological upset, and often are. We first point out the many physiologically based problems that can interfere with your child's school experience because in our rush to help our children, we often assume that we've done something wrong. As a consequence, we don't even look at other, equally likely possibilities that also need attention but that aren't psychologically based.

Often overlooked are physical problems. For instance, even with the physical screening tests performed annually in many schools, children's visual or hearing problems often go undetected. Any time a child performs at less than anticipated levels and isn't suffering an obvious or serious medical or psychological problem, vision and hearing screenings by medical professionals are warranted. Many children who underachieve or are labeled "problem" children, and who are subsequently evaluated by pediatric vision or hearing professionals, are found to have undetected problems with vision, hearing, or both. Such problems interfere with their learning, giving rise to frustration and often acting-out behaviors.

Even if a child is reevaluated for hearing and vision problems and is found to have none, other undiagnosed medical problems should be considered, especially if there is a history of problems that are hereditary (such as diabetes). Mild forms of a number of illnesses can easily cause inattention, concentration problems, difficulty with vision and hearing, and even behavior problems.

Some Typical Characteristics of Children with Learning Disorders

Children with learning disorders (LDs) may display a variety of traits including poor reading comprehension and poor spoken language, writing, and reasoning abilities. Other traits may include an assortment of symptoms of brain dysfunction, including uneven and unpredictable test performance, perceptual impairments, motor disorders, and emotional characteristics such as impulsiveness, low tolerance for frustration, and maladjustment. Hyperactivity, inattention, and distractibility may be associated with LDs, but they are not examples of LDs.

Although the presentation of a learning disorder may be subtle, its effect on your child's ability is not. Equally important, a child with undiagnosed LDs (some children have more than one) may be seen by teachers and other students as being merely unmotivated, lazy, or even stupid. It should come as no surprise, then, that many children seen as having behavioral problems are simply frustrated with their inability to learn effectively, regardless of the effort they expend. Tragically, because these children often go undiagnosed and untreated, they instead learn to accept the negative judgments of their teachers and peers, which in turn lead to poor self-esteem, depression, acting-out behaviors, and an overall feeling of incompetence. Learning disorders are treatable, but if they are not recognized and treated, a difficult course lies ahead for the child. A child who cannot learn basic math in grade school will not be able to learn geometry or algebra in high school. The learning of all subjects is hindered greatly in a child who has difficulty reading.

What Is a Learning Disorder?

According to the Individuals with Disabilities Education Act (formerly the Education of the Handicapped Act), a learning disorder is defined as a "disorder in one or more of the basic psychological processes involved in understanding or in using spoken or written language, which may manifest itself in an imperfect ability to listen, think, speak, read, write, spell or to do mathematical calculations." This definition includes reading disorder (dyslexia), brain injury, attention deficit hyperactivity disorder (ADHD), perceptual disorders, and developmental aphasia. It does not include people with mental retardation, students who have difficulty learning because of visual or hearing problems, children with behavior disorders, or children who are culturally, economically, or environmentally disadvantaged. Also required for diagnosis with an LD is a severe discrepancy between the child's potential (as measured by IQ testing) and his current status (as measured by achievement tests).

Learning disorders are thought to be neurologically based, making it difficult to identify the cause or causes. According to several studies, learning disorders affect about twenty percent of the population (although other research puts that percentage between two percent and three percent) and occur more often in boys than in girls at approximately a five-to-one ratio. Some studies cite an even higher ratio of seven-to-one. No race, religion, or cultural, social, or economic background is exempt. Equally important is that most children with learning disorders are bright children—some are even gifted. Having a learning disorder does not mean your child is not bright; it means only that he learns differently than other children, and that he can and will learn if provided with the proper academic resources. Early recognition and treatment are paramount to the child's success in school and later in adulthood.

Recognizing the Symptoms of a Learning Disorder

Often it is the parents who initially recognize that their child is not learning as she should. Observing preschool children of the same age, they may realize that their child cannot recite the alphabet, count to ten, remember her birth date, or put together a simple ten-piece puzzle—and that the child has neither the desire nor the inclination to learn. As the child enters school, she may complain of headaches or stomachaches every morning before school. In school, she may ask to see the nurse several times a day or ask to use the restroom—anything to avoid the schoolwork that she is having extreme difficulty learning. Sometimes, at this young age, these complaints are the only indication that something isn't right.

The slightly older child may have displayed early signs that her parents perceived to be those indicating a gifted child. By age two, she recites her name, address, and phone number. By three she begins to read on her own, is able to count to twenty, and is typing out the alphabet on the computer. She enters kindergarten, and her parents are surprised at the first parent-teacher conference to learn that their daughter cannot fit shapes into the proper spaces, that she scribbles or cannot color within the lines, and that she is unable to hold a pencil correctly.

An older child who has an average or above-average IQ and who is doing well in most subjects but is failing math and science, for instance, exhibits a discrepancy between his IQ (what he is capable of achieving) and what he is actually achieving. Sometimes a learning problem is subtle. A child may have excellent expressive language skills, but when assigned to write a short story, he struggles to write even a paragraph. Homework becomes a nightly battle—he forgets his school books, or he has no idea what the assignment is because he can't remember what he was told. Yet, the same child can recite historical dates and the names of all the presidents of the United States. All of these examples are warning signs that a child may have a learning problem or a learning disorder (not all learning problems are necessarily learning disorders; the child may just be slower in acquiring certain skills).

Warning signs of learning disorders include:

- Inability to understand and follow directions of more than one step

- Difficulty remembering what he was just told

- Lack of organizational skills

- Lack of coordination in playing sports, walking, holding a pencil, tying a shoelace

- Difficulty remembering: "I forget," "I don't remember," "I don't know."

- Problems conceptualizing time; confused by words like "yesterday," "tomorrow"

- Refusal to do homework

- Taking far too long to complete homework

- Daydreaming

- Wanting to be the boss and make own decisions

- Failure in schoolwork because of difficulty with reading, writing, and math skills

- Strong dislike for school

A child who consistently experiences any of these problems should be evaluated by a professional. First, however, a parent should consult with the child's teacher and ask some important questions, such as these: How does my son's work compare to his classmate's? In what areas does he have the most difficulties? How does he compare with his peers on standardized tests? Does she have difficulty paying attention in class? Is he impulsive? Is his work sloppy or neatly written? Is he the first to finish a test or one of the last? If he finishes last, is his work complete? Does she seem immature for her age? Has he expressed the belief that he can't do the work? Does she appear depressed? Answers to these types of questions will be valuable information to pass on to the mental health professional working with your child.

Reading Disorder

As we discussed in chapter four, reading disorder, popularly known as dyslexia, is distinguished by challenges in learning to read. Difficulties in learning to write, spell, speak, and to work with numbers are also often associated with this disorder.

According to the National Institutes of Health, children with reading disorder generally exhibit one or more of the following symptoms:

- Difficulty in learning and remembering the printed word

- Difficulty in writing

- Letter reversal (b for d, or p for q)

- Changed order of letters in words ("tac" for "cat") or numbers ("13" for "31")

- Persistent spelling errors

- Leaving out or interjecting words while reading

- Mistaking vowel sounds or substituting one consonant for another

- Delayed or inadequate speech

- Difficulty with choosing the right word when speaking

- Problems with direction (up and down, left and right)

- Problems with time (before and after)

- Clumsiness and awkwardness using hands

- Illegible handwriting

The exact cause of reading disorder is unknown. But most experts agree that a number of components (educational, psychological, and biological) presumably act in combination to cause the disorder. Therapy may be imperative to help the child conquer the emotional effects of reading disorder. The prognosis is good for children who are identified early, have good self-esteem, have the support of family and friends, and are involved in an appropriate remedial program of sufficient length.

Seeking Professional Help

It's difficult when you suspect that something isn't quite right, but to deny that there is a problem is only denying the services and interventions your child needs to feel good about herself, to succeed in school, and ultimately to succeed throughout the coming years.

It's important for the child to remember that he is not alone. Many children have some sort of learning disorder, as do adults (Thomas Edison, the inventor of the lightbulb, had multiple difficulties in school; Albert Einstein was labeled a slow learner). Fortunately today many professionals specialize in this area, and testing is available for children suspected of having a learning disorder.

The first step is to talk with the child's teacher and determine what type of testing is available through the school system—then to make arrangements for the testing. If the teacher is hesitant or does not think testing is necessary (but you do) send a letter to the principal requesting that your child be tested.

Your other option is to have your child tested privately through a clinic, a mental health center, a mental health professional in an independent or group practice, or a learning center. Referrals to specialists who conduct testing can be obtained from the school, from a family doctor, or from the child's pediatrician. Mental health professionals such as psychologists and learning specialists also assess learning disorders.

Typical testing and evaluation for learning disorders will include psychological testing, educational testing, and neuropsychological testing (which looks for neurological causes of psychological difficulty). A child may also be assessed by a language and speech pathologist, an audiologist (hearing specialist), and an ophthalmologist (vision specialist). A youngster may also be referred to a child psychiatrist if he is experiencing emotional problems—depression, for example, or poor self-esteem—and therapy may be indicated.

After it is established that a child has a learning disorder and after sessions with the parents, recommendations will be made for appropriate placement in school, special education, and speech-language therapy, if needed. The psychiatrist may prescribe medication if hyperactivity or distractibility are major concerns. The hyperactivity and distractibility may be the result of the child also having attention deficit hyperactivity disorder

(ADHD) comorbid (coexisting) with the learning disorder. In fact, if your child is diagnosed with a learning disorder and has not been evaluated for ADHD, we recommended that she be evaluated for this disorder because a sizable number of children with a learning disorder also have ADHD. Likewise, many children with ADHD also should be evaluated for learning disorders

Treatment for Learning Disorders

Remediation is always indicated for learning disorders. Remediation focuses on the most advantageous way to offset neurological inefficiencies that block the learning process of a fundamental academic or nonacademic ability. Sometimes, however, it is necessary for the child to be involved in psychological therapy before remediation begins. A child whose self-worth or self-esteem is so low that he sees himself as a complete failure (unable to master reading, for instance) must learn to feel better about himself before he is able to tackle the hard work involved in remediation. Although therapy may not be indicated for some children, a parent should keep in mind that this does not mean that a child has not suffered or will not ever suffer emotionally as a result of his learning disorder. All children with learning disorders suffer some emotional distress as a result of their inability to learn what others around them appear to learn so easily. Once deemed ready for remediation, the child is then able to believe in himself. He will have to work harder than the other children, but his boost in confidence will be noticeable. His frustration and fear of school will greatly diminish as he sees that he can learn and achieve success.

Keep in mind that psychotherapy is never enough for the learning disordered child, that sometimes remediation alone is enough, and that sometimes both remediation and psychotherapy are needed. Because parents' educational expectations must now be adjusted to the ability of the child, supportive therapy is often recommended not only to educate the parents about learning disorders, but also to help reduce any negativity in the home that arose out of frustration and misunderstanding. Individual therapy for learning disordered children with low self-esteem, aggressive behavior, tantrums, or lack of assertiveness is also recommended.

Children with learning disorders who attend public schools are entitled to special educational services in the least restrictive environment. Deficits in learning must be severe to qualify for services under the federal Public Law 101-479, the Individuals with Disabilities Education Act (IDEA); that is, the child must be at least two years behind her expected ability in one or more areas (for example, reading and math) to be eligible for an IEP (individualized educational program). Children who do not qualify for services under IDEA may be eligible for assistance under section 504 of the Rehabilitation Act of 1973.

Behavioral and Emotional Problems Seen in Children with Learning Disorders

As previously mentioned, children with learning disorders may have emotional problems as a consequence of their failure to achieve in one or several areas. Depression may be apparent, and parents may recognize the symptoms. But other children—children who just retreat quietly to their room—may go undetected. However, if retreating to the bedroom is unusual for the child, then parents must recognize that this is another symptom of depression.

Low self-esteem, demoralization, and social skills deficits are also associated with LDs. These children are often hurt and angry, confused by the fact that they seem so different from the other children around them without understanding why. They may have few friends due to their poor social skills. Feelings of insecurity may place them in the role of a helpless victim, or they may become bossy and controlling "know-it-alls." They often strive for independence, clearly wanting to live by their own set of rules. They want to establish a sense of control because they see their lives as being out of control.

The latter children often develop behavioral problems, acting out in unacceptable ways in school, in the home, and even in social situations. They may become aggressive with peers, parents, and teachers, run with the wrong crowd, and be uncooperative or oppositional. Professional intervention is highly recommended if the situation is out of control. Children with learning disorders have nearly a fifty percent chance of dropping out of school. Some children with a learning disorder also may have conduct disorder (CD), oppositional defiant disorder (ODD), attention deficit hyperactivity disorder (ADHD), or major depression.

Attention Deficit Hyperactivity Disorder

With the advent of the *DSM-IV*, attention deficit disorder (ADD) is now properly referred to as attention deficit hyperactivity disorder (ADHD), predominantly inattentive type. Some authorities on ADHD agree, saying ADD is nothing more than ADHD without the hyperactivity. Others feel that ongoing research will show ADD and ADHD to be two different disorders with subtle but important differences.

ADHD is one of the most common disorders diagnosed in childhood; at least one or two children in every classroom in the United States have ADHD. Although the estimates seem to vary, according to the *DSM-IV*, ADHD is found in three to five percent of school-aged children.

ADHD is a neurobiological disorder that exists in the brain and central nervous system. Its characteristic problems (tempering motion, mood swings, and paying attention) stem from neurobiological malfunctioning. It begins before age seven but may not be identified until the child is older. ADHD is characterized by age-inappropriate impulsivity, distractibility, inattention, and hyperactivity. Boys with this disorder often have behavioral problems and almost always are diagnosed at a much earlier age than girls. Girls often have underlying depression or anxiety, thus many may go undiagnosed and untreated.

As with many other disorders named before a complete appreciation of them had been reached, ADHD is a misnomer. There is no "deficit" in attention with ADHD. Instead, for most with ADHD, the largest problem is distractibility. Although those with ADHD can actually pay close attention, they seem to lack the physiological mechanism to consciously sustain attention to a particular subject or activity.

For instance, a child or adult without ADHD can choose to pay attention to a topic or activity even if he is not interested. A child or adult *with* ADHD, however, has difficulty sustaining focus on things he is not actively interested in, even if he consciously wants to. The environment presents myriad things to draw his attention; the resulting distractibility makes mastering schoolwork particularly hard, even though a large portion of ADHD people are quite bright. It's important that parents know that ADHD is not a learning disorder, although it is often referred to as such. Children with ADHD can learn, but distractibility interferes with their concentration, making learning more difficult. It is important to note that some children with ADHD do have a learning disorder.

However, ADHD does not affect just the child's ability to perform in an academic setting. It also plays havoc with the child's personal relationships with friends, classmates, parents, siblings, and teachers. In other words, ADHD affects the child in all aspects of his life.

Young children with ADHD often complain of boredom in a roomful of interesting toys, shifting from one toy to the next, not being able to sit and concentrate long enough to play with a particular toy. Quickly bored, they then move on to the next toy, or the stereo, or the electric outlets, or Mom's collection of crystal! They often move without thinking. For example, they may climb a bookcase without realizing that it could topple down: Their goal is to reach that interesting item on the top shelf. Their impulsivity usually gets them into a great deal of trouble. They may dart out into the street in their haste to pet the friendly dog who just emerged from the neighbor's house. In other words, they act first rather than think first.

Children with ADHD are easily distracted by tasks that are unimportant, but they often are extremely focused on activities they particularly enjoy (like playing electronic games, which are always stimulating). Unless engaged in a stimulating project, they are often unable to sit still in school or to concentrate. The school environment is often not stimulating enough to hold their attention.

Although some children with ADHD may have difficulty paying attention, staying seated, keeping their hands to themselves, and remaining quiet, others may be seen as spacey, often daydreaming or staring out the window. Children with ADHD are easily distracted by their environment. They hear the pencil drop in the back of the room, they see the squirrel running up the tree and the maintenance man walking past the classroom door. They are bombarded by stimuli, making it difficult for them to concentrate. That is why some children with ADHD will produce better work when a teacher is sitting or standing next to them—the teacher keeps them focused on their schoolwork.

Such children usually take longer to organize, to begin a task, and complete it than do other children—which means they often do not finish a test taken in the classroom because they run out of time. Homework is painfully and often carelessly completed and then is rarely turned in or is turned in late—usually because the children cannot remember where they put it. Organizing, following directions, and completing tasks are very difficult; they simply have too many thoughts vying for their attention at the same time, making it nearly impossible to select those thoughts that demand immediate and proper attention.

To understand these children, we must understand the disorder. ADHD can be viewed in many ways. The two main ways are both helpful for understanding this disorder. First, persons with ADHD may have minds that are very disinhibited, making concentration neurologically very difficult; or second, their minds do not "jump start" themselves, and they need constant stimulation to remain aware, let alone to focus. In either case, ADHD is not willful misbehavior, moral failing, or lack of trying. Rather, the inability of a child with ADHD to regulate her behavior is the result of neurological inefficiencies that are beyond the child's control. The frustrations of these children and people's reactions to the children's misbehavior cause their self-esteem to plummet. More than our censure, these children deserve our caring support and the attention of a trained mental health professional.

Diagnosing ADHD

Often a child's teacher is the first to recognize that a child is distractible or overly active for her age. However, teachers sometimes miss the quiet and cooperative child with ADHD because this child rarely causes any disturbance in school. She is seen as a good student who pays attention, when in fact, she is usually immersed in daydreaming and unable to focus on the lesson. If she is identified, it is usually years later when she is failing academically.

It is often difficult to diagnose ADHD in children under the age of four or five unless the symptom of hyperactivity is extreme. Because there are no laboratory tests that can be employed for clinical assessment, diagnosis at all ages is based primarily on the history provided by parents, grandparents, and baby-sitters. After the child is of school age, the assessing mental health professional is able to obtain feedback from the parents, the teacher, other caretakers, and the child, gaining a full clinical picture.

Before a diagnosis of ADHD is determined, it is important that other mental disorders be ruled out, including anxiety disorder and mood disorder, because these disorders typically arise around the same time symptoms of ADHD may begin to present themselves. It should be noted that children with low IQs may display symptoms of ADHD when placed in a grade that demands more intellectual capacity than they can muster. They become overwhelmed or bored, and they may act out to amuse themselves. Similarly, gifted children who are not placed in an intellectually challenging grade level may be bored by the lack of stimulation and challenge and may also exhibit signs of ADHD. In both cases, the signs of ADHD noted are without regard to whether the child actually *has* ADHD; if he or she does, then his symptoms will be exacerbated by the inappropriate grade placement.

Because symptoms are similar, the following should all be ruled out before a diagnosis of ADHD is given (see chapter four for the symptoms of ADHD):

- Underachievement in school due to a learning disorder

- Attention lapses caused by petit mal seizures

- A middle ear infection that causes an intermittent hearing problem

- Disruptive or unresponsive behavior due to anxiety or depression

Treatment of ADHD

Children with ADHD are usually treated with stimulant medication, such as Ritalin, Dexedrine, Cylert, or Adderall. Those children who do not respond well to stimulant medication are often treated with antidepressants (imipramine, Wellbutrin) or serotonin-specific receptor inhibitors (SSRIs) such as Prozac, Zoloft, Paxil, or Effexor, or a combination of medications. However, an effective course of treatment also includes behavior modification, emotional support, academic intervention, parent education, possibly psychotherapy for the child, and sometimes family therapy as well—especially if the child has emotional or severe behavioral problems that interfere with his life and that of his family. Other disorders often overlap with ADHD, such as oppositional defiant disorder, conduct disorder, learning disorders, and depression, all of which need to be recognized and treated if the child is to succeed academically and socially.

If a medically treated child continues to have difficulties, or if the medication appears not to be working, then parents should consult a child and adolescent psychiatrist. Some children are treated effectively by a pediatrician or a neurologist—usually these children have mild ADHD without any additional medical concerns—but if your child has behavioral or emotional problems, then you must seek the advice of a psychiatrist who can evaluate the whole child. Not only can a psychiatrist provide therapy and evaluate further for other disorders that may be present along with the ADHD, but also psychiatrists are medical doctors who have much experience and knowledge about the medications used to treat ADHD. They are also much more aware of the newest medications available to treat children.

Although medications, psychotherapy, cognitive-behavioral therapy, and sometimes social-skills training, parent-skills training, and academic interventions, have all been found to help children with ADHD, some treatments that have been recommended in the past have not been beneficial. The following treatments for ADHD have not been found to be effective: restricted diets, special colored glasses, eye training, chiropractic adjustment and bone realignment, medicines to correct problems in the inner ear, megavitamins, treatment for yeast infection, allergy treatments, and vitamin and mineral supplements.

If you believe that your child might have ADHD, an evaluation is clearly indicated. In fact, if you have any reason to believe that your child has a learning disorder or any medical or emotional condition that makes learning and school more difficult for her, an evaluation is imperative.

Many medical or emotional problems may present themselves as behavior problems, poor performance in school, and difficult behavior at home. Often children with these difficulties are seen as bad kids, slow learners, or behavior problems. Once labeled as such, the children become as aware of the label as are the adults who have labeled them. Sadly, even an inappropriate label tends to stick, and children, believing in the infallibility of adults, adopt that label as truth. The label often becomes self-fulfilling.

Because school is such an important part of your youngster's life, with a far-reaching effect on his future, anything that interferes with his effectiveness in school should be dealt with as soon as possible. The child will continue to fall behind, sometimes irreparably, until the problem is identified and treated.

Children Who Refuse to Go to School

Children who refuse to go to school or who complain that they are ill every morning are often suffering from a fear of school. This fear frequently begins in preschool or kindergarten and increases in severity until it finally crests around second grade. Parents, who usually have no idea why their child doesn't want to go to school, struggle to find the cause of their child's fear and anxiety. An unreasonable fear of school frequently follows a period when the child has spent a considerable amount of time growing closer to a parent at home (during summer recess or while a child is recovering from an illness, for example). This fear can also develop when the family has moved to a new school district or when the child has suffered the loss of a loved one or even the loss of a pet. Parents will witness a clinging behavior—the child often following a parent from room to room in the house. It's significant to make a distinction here: The fear is not of going to school, but of leaving the home! The fears are not unlike those seen in children with separation anxiety disorder (see chapter four).

Preteens and teenagers may have other reasons for refusing to attend school, including difficulty with peer relationships, academic underachievement, fear of performing in front of peers, and the fear of social situations. More than half of the children diagnosed with separation anxiety disorder have parents with anxiety or mood disorders. And most children (ninety-two percent) diagnosed with separation anxiety disorder also have a mood or anxiety disorder.

Children and teenagers with separation anxiety disorder, a mood disorder, school phobia, or a history of school absenteeism should be in individual therapy while receiving guidance from their parents. Sometimes family therapy is also indicated.

School Absenteeism

There may be many reasons for school absenteeism besides separation anxiety disorder, including other psychiatric disorders such as mood disorder, phobic disorder, obsessive-compulsive disorder, panic disorder, and psychotic disorders; also involved could be reasonable fear of bodily injury in an unsafe school environment, lack of parental cooperation regarding the importance of an education, substance abuse, or negative-modeling peers.

One of the most common types of school absenteeism is truancy in preadolescents and adolescents with conduct disorder. These children have no regard for authority and rules, and they are often quite active and aggressive. They may leave for school in the morning but never arrive, choosing instead to spend the day alone or with friends. Parents may not know that their children are not attending school until they receive a phone call, or they may not care if their children attend school because they believe an education is unimportant.

School absenteeism requires prompt professional intervention. The longer the child is out of school, the more complicated the picture becomes. The goals of intervention include setting limits, establishing a daily routine (providing structure), providing psychosocial intervention, gaining the cooperation of parents, and consulting with school officials. If these interventions do not produce results within two to four weeks, the therapist may prescribe antidepressant medication if an anxiety or mood disorder is indicated.

Seriously Disturbed Children

Children with emotional disturbances may be labeled "seriously emotionally disturbed," defined by the Individuals with Disabilities Education Act as "a condition exhibiting one or more of the following characteristics over a long period of time and to a marked degree, which adversely affects educational performance:

- "An inability to learn that cannot be explained by intellectual, sensory, or health factors

- "An inability to build or maintain satisfactory interpersonal relationships with peers and teenagers

• "A general pervasive mood of unhappiness or depression; or a tendency to develop physical symptoms or fears associated with personal or school problems."

Children with severe emotional or behavioral problems are not coping with their immediate environment. Behaviors and characteristics of children with emotional disturbances include:

• Performing academically below grade level

• Impulsivity, hyperactivity, short attention span

• Aggressive behavior toward teachers and peers (acting out, fighting)

• Self-injurious behavior (head-banging, lip-biting, creating lacerations with penknives, paper clips, or other sharp objects)

• Temper tantrums, poor coping skills, crying spells (not age-appropriate)

• Excessive fears and anxieties

• Failure to initiate interaction with others, withdrawal from social interaction

Children with the more serious emotional disturbances (psychosis or schizophrenia) exhibit:

• Sharp mood swings

• Bizarre behavior

• Disordered thinking

• Excessive anxiety

Public schools provide individual educational programs (IEPs) for children with disorders, including those who are seriously emotionally disturbed. The goal is to assist children with academics, social skills, self-control, and self-esteem. Behavior modification (using positive reinforcement) is used to reduce behavior problems—a technique widely used for children with emotional-behavioral disorders—helping children to control their behavior and take responsibility for their actions. Behavior modification teaches children the cause and effect of inappropriate behavior by providing consequences for their actions and by rewarding appropriate behavior (earning tokens to gain privileges, for instance, or receiving praise, such as a hug for the younger child).

Although the IEP addresses an appropriate and free public school education for the child, it does not address therapy, which is frequently needed for the child with emotional/behavioral disturbances. Therapy, which is available from public or private mental health professionals, is coordinated with the parents, teachers, and any other mental health professionals working with the child, under the direction of the psychiatrist or psychologist.

Children of Divorce in the School Setting

A child's teachers should be told about a pending divorce. Just as you are helping to make the crisis and the inevitable transition easier on your child within the home, a child's teacher can also help support and encourage the child in the classroom with warmth and assurance. Keep in touch with teachers and school counselors and attend as many school functions as possible. School staff can alert you to any unusual behaviors your child might be experiencing in school due to the amount of stress he may be encountering. It takes approximately two years, according to experts, for a child to adjust to changes in the family structure—by then he should be performing equally to other children in school who have not had to make the transition to a single-parent home.

Students at High Risk

Some students are at a higher risk of dropping out of school than their peers. These include children with behavioral, learning, or emotional difficulties, children with high stress levels in the home, or those who have failed a grade, are involved with substance abuse, have been abused, suffer from low self-esteem, are facing pressures from the family (family dissolution), have expectations to make money or to care for certain family needs rather than finish school, or who are facing an untimely pregnancy. A consultation with a mental health professional may be needed.

There are many other reasons a child may not be excelling in school besides those mentioned in this chapter. It is impossible to define all of those reasons, but as you continue to read this book, keep this in mind: Any stressful special circumstances in the home such as a sibling with a disability, a parent with emotional or psychiatric problems, or any illness of the child can make it difficult for a child to perform at grade level. The informed parent looks at all areas in the child's life as possible reasons for struggles in school, keeping in mind that factors in the classroom may also be exacerbating the child's difficulties. As the child's parent, you are your child's best, and sometimes only, advocate. If your child is struggling, it behooves you both to find the source of that struggle.

SEVEN

When Bad Things Happen to Good Children

Occasionally circumstances arise in which children are exposed to unusual or particularly trying events. Parents file for divorce, tornadoes hit communities, earthquakes destroy, friends become ill, relatives die, siblings are born or adopted, fathers or mothers lose their jobs, financial problems develop, families move, robberies occur, and accidents happen. Any one of these circumstances may have a detrimental effect on a child, often leading to serious mental problems, especially depressive illness. The stress or depression, anger, hostility, shame, fear, and guilt—the negative feelings that can develop—are the result of the incident and the child's reaction to the incident. Often, during the aftermath of a discrete event, the child may deny any "bad" feelings or problems. Careful evaluation of the child by a competent professional will often reveal, however, long-term negative effects related to the event. Most frequently, depressive symptoms and behavioral changes offer the most revealing insight to the level of disturbance caused by the child's experience.

So how do you know whether your child is coping adequately with your pending divorce? Or whether your son is jealous of the new baby, or that your daughter feels she is the cause of Grandpa's death because she once wished him dead? Children often have difficulty communicating their feelings, because, unlike most adults, they have not yet mastered how to express their thoughts and emotions in words. If a child feels overwhelmingly angry, for instance, but lacks the vocabulary to express that anger, he may physically act out by displaying troublesome or even unacceptable behavior, such as physical or verbal aggression or both. Because children have different feelings, thoughts, behaviors, and coping mechanisms at different ages, parents frequently must determine what is appropriate at one age but inappropriate at another. This task becomes even more difficult when behaviors are the aftereffect of unique circumstances. This chapter will identify some universal events that are stressful for children and discuss some typical responses that are seen when a child's life is suddenly thrown off balance.

In the great majority of cases, clinically substantial depression is the primary diagnostic category. Far less frequently, but still significant in incidence, posttraumatic stress disorder (PTSD)—a result of severe emotional insult—can represent a serious therapeutic challenge, often requiring lengthy treatment.

Adjustment disorders are lower-order disruptions of emotional health and can also be caused by the types of events and situations listed earlier. Although not nearly as important as a cause of long-term disability in children, they are deserving of notice and treatment.

Separation anxiety disorder can also be occasioned by some of the events mentioned earlier. Usually transient when dealt with sympathetically and promptly, it can, nevertheless, represent a serious impediment to growth and maturation if ignored, or worse, if treated with disdain by parents. Recognition is the first important step to ensuring that this not-infrequent result of parental absence (however brief and insignificant to the parent), the death of a favorite pet, the hospitalization of a loved grandparent, or similar separation receives the attention it warrants.

When Bad Things Happen to Children

First, it is important to remember that each child reacts differently to stress. A child's age, temperament, personality, ability to understand, the immediate support received or not received from loved ones, and the child's relationship with her parents will all play a part in how a child reacts to stressful events. The manner in which parents react to the event—whether the parents were involved or the child was solely affected—may increase or decrease the amount of pressure the child experiences. Children who have a close, trusting parental relationship frequently handle stressful events much better than children who do not. When an older child experiences a special bond with her parents she is more apt to share her feelings without fear of being rejected. This trust and acceptance between parent and child permit the child to turn to a parent for help (and for comfort) during a crucial time even when the child is unable to express herself adequately. Such behavior is seen, for example, in a younger independent child who suddenly becomes fearful and clings to a parent. Parents who communicate with their children on a daily basis—listening to their hopes and fears—not only build a trusting relationship with their children, but also show them that they are a loved, accepted, and important member of the family. Building a strong relationship with your child also means that you are competent to recognize changes in behavior and in speech patterns—the signs that demonstrate that your child is facing a crisis.

Remember that a crisis is something that happens unexpectedly. But as parents we can prepare for some crises ahead of time. Some of the first steps we've just discussed: building a trusting relationship with your child, knowing and understanding your child's normal behavior so you are capable of recognizing changes, being available to talk and listen unconditionally, and demonstrating your love not only in words but also in actions.

Separation and Divorce

Without a doubt, separation and divorce are devastating events for adults (even for the spouse who wants out of the marriage). A separation, and ultimately a divorce, signals the end of a marriage and the end of the present family unit. As stressful and frightening as it is for the adults involved, it is far more stressful and frightening for the children. As adults we have the ability to look ahead. Even if we are fearful of the future, even if we have not been through a previous divorce, we understand what is happening and where we are headed. We understand, for instance, that one or both spouses will be moving from the marital home. But we also know that in the end everyone will have a place to live. We understand that our standard of living will change, that we will have less money, but we know that we will survive. We have an idea of the road ahead.

To children, however, divorce is an unknown road. Children live in the "now" and lack the maturity and understanding to look ahead to the future. Children, until they hit a certain level of maturity, understand only that Mom and Dad will not be living together. They don't understand why! They are incapable of understanding that a mother's drinking problem or a father's infidelity has led to the breakdown of the marriage.

Most older children today are aware of what it means for parents to be separated or divorced. They have friends or classmates whose parents are no longer living together. One of the greatest fears that our children experience is that they may lose one or both of their parents. In fact, some children have such a fear of losing their parents that they worry, sometimes unnecessarily, that their parents will divorce. If it can happen to other children, it can happen to them, they reason. Children don't want to believe or to accept that Mom and Dad will no longer be living together with them in the same house. Through the years, even after one or both parents have remarried, children will still secretly harbor the hope that Mom and Dad will remarry.

A pending divorce is a crisis both for parents and for children. Children will experience a wide range of emotions during this time. Even those children who are old enough to understand are confused and frightened as their security is threatened. Understandably, they worry about a whole range of issues: where they will live, what school they will attend, if they'll lose their best friend, or if their dog will continue to live with them. Children may also worry about which parent they will live with and whether they'll be able to remain in contact with the other parent. If Dad is the one moving from the marital home, they may express their desire to live with Dad "so he won't be alone," not realizing that Mom would then be the one alone. Their concerns invite fears of abandonment even before the separation takes place.

Some children may hold feelings inside, becoming sullen and depressed. Other children may suddenly become "perfect" children, believing that if their behavior is exemplary their parents will reconcile. And still other children may act out in an attempt to refocus their parents' attention from the separation and divorce issues to their misbehavior. Many children will carry feelings of guilt, believing that they are somehow to blame for their parents' separation. Children who become perfect or who act out often feel it is their responsibility to reunite Mom and Dad even if it means they must sacrifice themselves. But keep in mind that some children are not adversely affected. Some children do adjust and move on successfully, especially when Mom and Dad are able to keep the best interests of the children in mind at all times.

Parents who emotionally withdraw from their children during a pending divorce, who openly engage in verbal or physical warfare, who use the children as pawns by attempting to alienate the children from the other parent, or who involve the children in the dispute by confiding in or seeking comfort from the children leave children susceptible to physical and mental illness. The loving, conscientious, concerned parent worries about the impact of the divorce on his children.

With this in mind, in most cases divorce is one crisis that parents can prepare for. There is no point in talking with children about the "possibility" of a divorce. But after a divorce is certain, after the papers have been filed, parents should then talk together with their children, emphasizing that although the marriage is ending, their role as parents remains—they will both still love the children and continue to be their parents but they will do that from two households now, rather than one. Children should not be told the details of the divorce, nor should they be coerced, or bribed with promises or gifts, into taking sides.

The children's well-being is paramount—their best interests must come first, or we risk their physical and emotional health. Not all situations are ideal, however, so parents must draw on their own inner strengths to protect their children—not an easy task in some cases. Unfortunately there are parents who deliberately try to hurt or get even with the other parent, making life extremely difficult for the other parent and the children. A father who is abusive toward a mother, a mother who puts down the father to the children, or a parent who refuses visitation, often succeeds only in teaching children how to be abusive, causing a great deal of emotional stress for the children. Therefore, parents must make every effort to protect the children from witnessing struggles over material items, ugly conversations, and custody battles. These hateful battles are often more than children can manage.

So how does a parent know if the child needs therapy to help him through the transition? Look for changes in behavior that are troublesome and persistent, lasting for more than two weeks. Some signs include:

- Any acting-out behavior such as aggressive behavior toward parents, siblings, or peers at home, in school, or both; unusual or prolonged temper tantrums; stealing; truancy; breaking curfews; et cetera

- Depression (irritability, persistent crying, changes in sleeping habits, changes in appetite, nightmares, clinging behavior, fear of being left alone or other fears that are not age appropriate, withdrawing from family and friends, lack of interest in things the child normally enjoys)

- A decline in school grades due to the inability to concentrate

- Regression in previously learned skills (for instance, bed-wetting)

Because most parents are concerned about how the divorce will affect their child, many will seek the advice of a therapist on how best to help their child through this transition. Often one visit to a therapist is all that is necessary. By establishing this link with a mental health professional, parents will have someone to turn to if the need arises. Should your concerns persist, your child should be evaluated by a professional. If the therapist has concerns, short-term therapy may be recommended.

Illness or Death of a Parent

The illness of an immediate family member, or even of an important extended family member such as a much-loved grandparent, aunt, or uncle, can be terrifying for a child. She hears the concern of adults around her in muted tones and notes that conversations about the ill person cease when she walks into the room.

Although the serious illness of any loved family member is a trial for a child, a very ill parent can be emotionally devastating. Unarmed with the sophisticated knowledge that we as adults can use to understand another's illness, a child facing the prospect of the parent's removal to the hospital or actual presence there can suffer anxiety about separation or abandonment. Although a very young child may not possess the ability to appreciate the finality of death, the sense of imminent loss can be frightening, as can the sight of an ill, exhausted parent lying in a hospital bed. Chronic illness experienced by a loved adult can have a major impact on the child, especially if the loved one is a parent on whom the child depends. Without the ability to understand what is happening, or could happen, the child suffers a great deal of stress whether openly or privately.

A child's reaction to the illness or death of a family member differs from that of an adult. For very young children, death is seen as temporary—the typical cartoon character may die several times in the span of thirty minutes. By age five, until the age of nine or so, children begin to understand death but still not in the same manner as adults—they accept that death exists but willingly admit it could never happen to them or someone they know. Until children have a concept of death as a finality, they may express little emotion, although they witness and acknowledge that others are sad and upset. During these young years, most children believe that death happens only to old people. Even in adolescence, youth have not accepted that they themselves could actually die, even if they have lost a peer or a sibling.

Around age seven, children begin to have questions about death—showing what may appear to be extraordinary concern—worrying excessively that one of their parents might die. One mother, who found her child crying in bed shortly after tucking him in, said her son was crying because he was worried that after he married and had children, everyone he knew would have died and there would be no one around to take care of him, "not even you and Daddy." Although her concern was appropriate, this mother had no cause for alarm—we can expect a child around the age of seven or eight to take a normal and predictable interest in dying, death, funerals, cemeteries, and funeral cars, even if he has never known anyone who has died.

Emotions expressed after the death of a parent, then, depend on the age and developmental level of the child. Although it would appear that the death of a parent would cause an unlimited number of problems for the child during this time and well into the future, studies have shown that this is not necessarily the case. What can actually become more problematic for the child is the behavior of the surviving parent before and after the death of the spouse. The unavailability of a surviving grief-stricken parent can be confusing to the child and may cause the child to feel the loss of two parents—not just one. A parent who is unavailable emotionally often has a greater impact on the young child than does the loss of the deceased parent. As long as there is available a supportive adult (grandparent, aunt, uncle, for example) who meets the child's emotional and physical needs, answers questions, and attends to the child, she is less prone to feel abandoned.

Infants experience the loss of the parent and exhibit the loss by withdrawing, crying more than normal, and even making facial expressions. By the age of two, children know that their security has been annihilated, but they may appear unaffected. Yet we know they have shut down—unintentionally denying their feelings, because they do not have the ability to communicate. Other children will act out. We will witness behavioral changes such as the child becoming too demanding, throwing tantrums, experiencing nightmares, and clinging to the surviving parent or a favored blanket or stuffed animal. In many children we find some degree of regression—suddenly they can no longer feed themselves or even put on their socks.

Children who have a general understanding of death usually show their grief in one of two ways: They either immediately react and grieve, or they persist in the belief that the family member is still alive (children may be found searching for the parent in the rooms of the house associated with the deceased parent). Grief may be ventilated off and on for several weeks, frequently erupting at unexpected moments. Children should be encouraged to express their grief unreservedly with the support of their loved ones close by. When a surviving parent is not available to the child, other relatives or friends should be. If those closest to the child are struggling to cope with their own emotions, crisis intervention therapy is available for bereavement issues.

Because older children are still dependent on their parents, they, too, may regress and display helplessness, powerlessness, or childish actions. Sometimes, however, they just continue on as if nothing has happened. The adults closest to them may feel that the children really don't care or haven't been affected by the loss. These children, like those just described, need help in expressing their feelings.

Most children are resilient, but the surviving parent or a relative should monitor a child closely, watching for continuing signs of denial, depression, falling grades in school, and behavior that a parent is not able to handle. If you know your child is still experiencing difficulties months later, after you've made repeated attempts to encourage the child to talk about the pain she feels, then the child needs outside, professional intervention. In fact, in one study where bereavement psychotherapy continued for eight weeks for children between the ages of seven and eleven, the results showed a decrease in depression, emotional turmoil, and behavior disturbances compared with a waiting list control group.

Lastly, a parent should never attempt to spare the child from the knowledge of an impending death of a parent or other close relative or friend. A parent who cannot express and share feelings with her child (who already knows something is wrong) shows by example that this subject is not to be discussed. Parents who cannot talk with their child will benefit greatly by talking with a professional for guidance. Shortly after a parent or other loved one passes away, an adult family member must tell the child what has happened, stressing that everyone is upset but that all family members will pull together and help each other during this difficult time.

Family Moves

It is rare that a family remains in the same house from the time their first (or only) child is born to the time their last child completes high school. A job relocation may send a family from one end of the country to the other, or a raise may provide the family with the opportunity to purchase a larger home across town. Either way, it means uprooting and leaving behind everything that is familiar and trading it for the unknown.

Moving is a stressful event for all family members, but especially for children who have already entered school. For children, moving to a new location means leaving behind old friends, making new friends in a school where everyone else already has a best friend, and establishing themselves in an unfamiliar school. It means adjusting to new circumstances, new routines, and new people.

Adolescents usually do not want to move. They may beg to be left behind with a relative or a friend, even when the move is to a new area that offers a variety of novel activities and exciting places to visit. This is because their peer group is everything to them at this point in their lives. They are of the age when they are moving away from parental dependency and are seeking their own identity. Their friends are now their confidants and often their role models. To have to form new relationships as the "new kid on the block" can be frightening and stressful. For this reason many mental health professionals advise that teenagers who are in their senior year of high school be permitted to stay behind either with a relative or trusted friends.

It is best to announce the move and explain the reasons for it: "The only way Dad is able to keep his job is if he accepts this transfer, so together we hope to make this a very exciting opportunity for all of us." Although we advise that many family matters are best explored in family meetings with input from all members, if the move *must* be made, then it cannot be voted upon. But all children should have the opportunity to discuss the move and provide their input without parents becoming critical. Parents do best by acknowledging their children's feelings.

As the move is being planned, encourage your children to take part in some of the decision making—from making travel arrangements to packing to deciding how to transport the family pet. If affordable, permit children to travel with you when you look for a new house. While there, tour the city and drive by schools, libraries, shopping centers, movie theaters, beaches or ski areas, and the typical teenage hangouts. If taking the children with you is not an option, have them write for information from the chamber of commerce to learn more about the new location. Subscribe to the city's newspaper before moving—they can read about local events.

Although moving across town can be just as upsetting as moving to another state, when a move is across town children should be told that their friends are welcome to visit—that the move does not mean they have to give up their friends.

Obviously the most telling sign of stress is depression—before and after the move. Remember that it is natural for children who are leaving friends behind to feel depressed. However, when the depression becomes disabling and persists, parents must seek the advice of a mental health professional. Referrals may be obtained from neighbors, employees, school personnel, mental health association, the American Academy of Child and Adolescent Psychiatry (see the appendices for contact information), a local hospital, your new doctor, or even your new dentist. A move is particularly stressful when a family is moving away from their relatives and friends. A psychiatrist or other mental health professional can offer advice for all family members.

Natural Disasters

Some situations are completely out of a parent's control—situations that, due to the forces of nature, leave families homeless and without adequate food, clothing, medication, drinking water, and financial resources. The family environment collapses when tornadoes, earthquakes, mudslides, fires, and hurricanes strike. The emotional and physical consequences can be devastating for all family members but even more so for the children, who are emotionally vulnerable.

After a disaster, it is understandable that children will be frightened. The actual event was frightening in itself, but they may have also witnessed the death or injury of a family member or friend. Their fears are normal, especially their fear of abandonment.

Parents' first concern is to care for their children. They must provide for their physical needs, including food, shelter, and medical care, and immediately respond to the children's emotional needs. The Federal Emergency Management Agency (FEMA) has these recommendations:

- Listen to what your child is saying (or not saying) regarding what has happened; clarify facts when necessary; some children may need to be encouraged to talk because they may be bewildered by the events; parents should not be afraid to express some of their own concerns while assuring children that they will continue to care for them

- Although it may be tempting to separate your family members by removing them from the disaster area to the homes of others, this may only increase the anxiety levels of some children who may fear that their parents may not come back for them; children's greatest need at this time is to know they are safe with their parents

- Permit children to assist in the cleanup process; even young children can help after a disaster, if directed; as the process continues, children can then see that things are beginning to return to normal; point out how everyone is pitching in to clean up the area to make it better for all

- Explain to children why it is necessary for the family to move to an emergency shelter; let them know that many other families might also be staying there and that more than likely, people will be sleeping on the floor in sleeping bags and that you will be staying there until you are either able to return to your home or until you find another home to live in; because children will feel that they have lost complete control of their lives, they should be encouraged to help locate a spot in the shelter where the family will live temporarily and to place sleeping bags on the floor in the family's space

- Although the demands on adults are great at this time, children still need to play; usually the American Red Cross, another similar community organization, or private citizens will provide toys, educational materials, and group activities for children

- As an adult you will have much to do, but your children will require much more of your time than usual whether it's just to sit and talk with them, take a walk, play a card game, or hold and comfort them

- Remain calm and in control; assure your children that you are doing everything humanly possible to protect and care for them; discipline with firm limits and be consistent; some acting-out behaviors and emotional up and downs are normal

Usually crisis intervention therapists are sent to the disaster site to help victims of all ages deal with the trauma. Even if your child appears to be doing well, always take advantage of these free counseling services. These therapists are specially trained to counsel victims of disaster.

Children tend to hold back initially after a disaster, and their needs and demands may then affix to other problems. If any of the following symptoms persist weeks or even months after the disaster, seek professional help for your child:

- Continued fear that the disaster will strike again

- Trouble concentrating

- Excessive worrying

- Signs of helplessness

- Nightmares or trouble sleeping

- Clinging behavior

- Irritability

- Excessive crying

- Fear of being left alone or being separated from parents for even short periods

- Persistent insecurity

- Feelings of immortality (teens)

- Reckless behaviors (teens)

Posttraumatic stress disorder (PTSD) is a result of severe stress in the environment. Its long-lasting behavioral and emotional consequences appear after a child has been involved in, been witness to, or received news of a shocking event that affected a family member or a friend. The event may be the result of a natural disaster, child molestation, war, an airplane crash involving a loved one, or any other traumatic event experienced or witnessed by the child. The child is left feeling defenseless and apprehensive and may experience any of the following:

- A fear of being separated from their parents

- A fear of their own death

- Fear of future injury

- Nightmares

- Somatic symptoms

- Anxiety, depression

- Guilt that they survived or were not injured

- Guilt that they were unable to save someone

- Self-blame, believing that they somehow caused the event

- Regression of prior developmental milestones

- Reenactment of the situation in play or behavior

Individual therapy encompasses engaging in play and fantasy, drawing, telling stories, reassessing the event, giving instructions to the child on how to cope, and bolstering the child's self-esteem. Sometimes group therapy is employed.

The Blessed Event

Most parents are thrilled to learn that they are going to have a baby. Most children are just as excited—until reality sets in. Perhaps one of the greatest concerns of parents is how their first child will feel about the addition of another child. How will we tell him? they ask each other. How will she feel? How can we best prepare him for a new brother or sister? Will she be jealous?

And perhaps the greatest fear is that the first child will suddenly feel unloved as she watches the amount of attention that is heaped on the new baby, from the wonderful brightly colored presents to the new items in the nursery to Grandma and Grandpa rushing over to see the new baby.

We cannot say for certain how your child will react, because much depends on his temperament. Many children are excited to learn that a new baby will be "moving in," and that excitement never wanes. Other children are initially excited but after the first week or so want to know when the baby will be returning to the hospital—and they're not asking because they are going to miss their new sibling! They've had enough and now want things to return to normal. This is normal because they once received all of your attention, and now it seems that the baby is receiving what should be coming to them. A minority of children, although initially excited, lose interest quickly and become extremely jealous to the point that their behavior, their words and actions, clearly indicate anger. When such a child becomes stuck at this stage, and the anger continues—anger that may be directed at you and also at the baby—for more than a few weeks, professional intervention may be indicated. Talk with your doctor first about your child's behavior and his jealousy.

Financial Stress and Strife between Parents

Very important, regardless of the age of your child, is how the family deals with financial stress and with strife between the parents. Dealt with effectively, these concerns can actually add strength to the emerging adult; dealt with poorly, they can rob your child of his ability to handle stress, frustration, and anger. The way parents handle these concerns provides a model that the child can internalize as the proper way to handle financial difficulty and interpersonal conflict, especially with a spouse.

Unfortunately, and perhaps unfairly, the types of situations you must handle as an adult and the way in which you handle them will most likely have long-term effects on the way your child sees the world (either as a safe place that he can handle, come what may; or as a dangerous place, one that is too powerful for him to deal with, a place where he must simply accept the whims of fate and suffer accordingly).

Although as adults it's easy for us to relate to the worry we experience about financial problems, our children have neither our maturity nor our experience to mediate that worry. Your worry and concern can be a fearful matter for your child to witness. He may see himself as the cause of your financial distress and feel guilty and "bad." Your struggle may then become his struggle. Without your resources of maturity and experience, he can be easily overwhelmed and become depressed.

Although we are not suggesting that children be kept entirely in the dark regarding family financial problems, we *are* suggesting that continual comments about the family's lack of financial resources serve no purpose but to worry the children with something they can do little about. If Dad has lost his job and may be unemployed for several months, it's all right to have a family meeting and explain that the "family needs to cut back on spending for a while, until things get back to normal" and to ask children for ways they can think of to help (not badgering for junk food in the grocery store, demanding unneeded toys or $100 shoes, et cetera).

What's most important to remember is that the way you handle problems, seek solutions, and resolve difficulties has a major impact on your child. His ability to cope with problems as an adult will be learned from you.

Child Abuse

Child abuse is the repeated mistreatment or neglect of a child by a parent, baby-sitter, relative, friend, or other adult. The abuse may be physical (burning, beating, slapping, failing to provide adequate food, clothing, and shelter), emotional (omission of caring, warmth, concern; lack of supervision), sexual (incest, rape, or other sexual activity between an adult and the child), or verbal (inordinate amount of shouting, demeaning or beleaguering the child). In all cases it harms or injures the child.

Child abuse can occur in any family and can involve one or both parents. The effects of child abuse are severe, leading to emotional or physical disabilities and even death. Children who are abused may become acting-out adolescents or adults engaging in violent or criminal activities and other antisocial behaviors. They may even continue the cycle of abuse with their own children or spouse.

Child abuse is most often triggered by overpowering parental stress over a situation that needs to be resolved. It is commonly a reaction to previous or present-day problems or pressures that parents cannot cope with, such as drug or alcohol problems, an inferior self-image, unmet emotional needs, lack of parenting knowledge, unsatisfactory childhood experiences, social isolation, unrealistic expectations, and frequent crises. If financial concerns are considerable or if a marital relationship is in serious trouble, a parent may verbally attack the child out of frustration. Or a child with severe behavioral problems, undiagnosed and untreated, may be physically abused by an isolated, frustrated, critical parent who has finally reached the end of her rope. Troubled families need immediate treatment. Mental health workers, such as social workers, and supportive friends and relatives can help families live together and cope with the crisis. Sometimes all a parent needs is a supportive someone to talk with or a friend or relative to relieve him a few hours a week so he can spend time away from the child. Most abusive parents are lucid, that is, they are not mentally ill. They are able to master parenting effectively and learn to think better of themselves with knowledge and guidance.

Abuse that has been ongoing—such as the alcoholic parent who consistently beats the children or the critical parent who consistently belittles the child for not acting like an adult—demands professional treatment. Long-term therapy for children and parents is essential and is often needed to stop the cycle of abuse. Abusive parents who lack the knowledge and ability to raise a child must be taught appropriate parenting skills and interventions. They must also learn the stages of childhood development when they can't understand the child's needs and behaviors. How to set realistic expectations and how to handle crisis situations without losing control are also goals in therapy.

The Child with a Long-Term Illness
A child with a chronic illness risks acquiring related psychological problems as he tries to cope with the knowledge that his illness is not going to go away. Mental health professionals who

work with these children say almost all of them initially reject the idea that anything is wrong with them that can't be treated. After acceptance occurs, indignation and blame follow.

A young child may blame himself, believing that something he did wrong caused the illness. Thus the child may view his illness as a punishment for any number of "wrongful" deeds. Often parents, doctors, or other caretakers are blamed for the illness. It's not unusual for the child to become angry at his parents or doctors for not finding a cure. Dietary restrictions, inability to participate in typical childhood activities, and numerous discomforting treatments may induce detachment and bitterness toward life and other people. The child may resent the attention and caring he receives and react negatively toward the coddling, or "babying," as some children describe it. Teenagers, on the other hand, recognize the necessity of relying on others for assistance. However, it becomes increasingly difficult for them because they are of the age when they are struggling to achieve independence and trying to form their own identity. Whatever the age of the child, she should be given as much information about her illness as she is capable of understanding.

Children with chronic long-term illnesses may experience academic setbacks, or in some cases, school avoidance issues may become a problem—both of which generate feelings of loneliness and of being different from peers—at a time when children particularly need contact with friends. Parents should make every effort not to overly protect the child. Like any other child, he must learn to socialize and separate from the family.

A child who has a chronic illness is frequently treated by a team of specialists. This team often includes a child and adolescent psychiatrist, who should be kept up to date on the child's emotional status. Anytime a family is dealing with the stress of caring for an ill child, all members of the family are also affected. Caring for an ill child is stressful and often requires the intervention of a mental health professional who can teach parents better ways of coping with the pressures that are inherent.

Parents with Mental Illness

Compared to other children, a child with a parent who has a mental illness is at great risk for acquiring a mental illness himself. According to the American Academy of Child and

Adolescent Psychiatry, the risk is greater when the parent has bipolar disorder, schizophrenia, alcoholism, or major depression. When both parents have a mental illness, the risk is greatest.

Besides the obvious genetic risk, other risks include an uncertain family environment, inadequate parenting skills, absence of love and guidance from parents, and the parents' moods and behavior. But individual or family psychiatric treatment can help the child toward wholesome development. Factors that can decrease risks for the child include a secure attachment to a healthy adult, friends, school success, good coping skills, extracurricular activities, unfluctuating environment in her home, knowing that she is not to blame for the illness of the parent, and feeling loved by the ill parent.

The Adopted Child

Although there is nothing "bad" or "unexpected" about the fact that a child is adopted, we need to say a few things about the adopted child. Historically it has been believed that all adopted people have problems, if not as children then certainly as adults. Although it is true that some adopted children do have difficulties dealing with the realities of their status, most children do not. Overall, adopted children do just as well as nonadopted children in school, at home, and with peers.

It's imperative that the child be told that he was adopted. Unfortunately, there are two schools of thought here: One is that the child should be told at a very young age of his adoption; the other is that the child should not be told until he is old enough to understand. We believe that a child should be told at a very young age that he was adopted. In fact, we believe that the word "adopted" or "adopt" should be dropped into conversations occasionally (not frequently). A good way to introduce adoption is by using a photo album with the two- or three-year-old child. You can say such things as, "This is the family you lived with before we adopted you" (if the child was in foster care for even a few days after birth), or "We waited to adopt a baby for a long time. See how happy we are in this picture. This is the day we brought you home from the hospital." When "adopted" or "adopt" is used like this, a child never remembers being told that he was adopted. As the child matures, you can find many excellent books about adoption to read to him. We encourage parents to read these books to their children. They can be found in any library or bookstore.

Through the years, it's important that parents answer their children's questions about adoption truthfully. If you do not know the answers, say so. Never lie about the child's birth family. A young child should not be told the circumstances surrounding his adoption until he is old enough to understand all of the dynamics involved. Usually this will not happen until the child is in his teen years. But always assess the maturity of the child before relaying the facts and providing pictures. Remember not to speak ill of the birth family, because it will make the child only suspicious. Even in the worst of situations, there is always something good that can be told about the birth parents. ("Your birth mother was very pretty, just like you.")

Don't believe that the child who doesn't ask questions isn't interested. With a child who appears uninterested, parents should continue to make reference to her adoption. You can do this easily. For instance, when a child has just accomplished a major feat, don't be afraid to say, "Your birth parents would have been so proud of you if they could have seen you today." Sometimes a child may think you do not want to discuss her adoption, so she doesn't ask questions for fear of hurting your feelings. Unfortunately, some adoptive parents don't want to discuss the topic because they are insecure, and the child picks up on this. If you are having difficulty addressing adoption with your child, please seek professional help.

Remember that it is normal for your child to have questions, so don't be offended. And he does have a right to any information you have available. A child who becomes so hung up on the adoption that he or she is having difficulty in school or at home should be seen by a mental health professional who understands what the child is experiencing. Any adoption agency in your area should be able to refer you to a professional who works with adopted children.

In Conclusion

It's important to remember that during family difficulties, some children noisily demand attention (and most often receive it). Other children, when stressed by circumstances they do not fully understand, become quiet and withdrawn, almost blending in with the background. They may act out in school, confide in friends, but at home they may work hard to be invisible to keep from being drawn into a conflict or circumstance they find overwhelming. Both the demanding child and the withdrawn child are signaling for help.

Even if your child seems unaffected by serious problems being experienced in your home, it is to your child's advantage to have at least a meeting or two with an experienced mental health professional to evaluate how he is really handling the family's distress. Children can sometimes be profoundly depressed yet appear "fine" to their already overwhelmed parents.

Remember that bad things happen to good people all the time. The difference between a permanently crippled life and a temporarily painful circumstance is recognition, then effective treatment.

EIGHT

Other Faces of Children: Fear, Anxiety, and Anger

Throughout life, from infancy to old age, we all experience fears, anxieties, and anger. Although these emotions are normal, if your child displays them to a disruptive extreme, they may alert you to underlying problems that should be addressed by a mental health professional. Here, we offer strategies for dealing with these common problems on your own and advice about when outside help may be warranted.

Fearful or Anxious Children

Not surprisingly, the fears and anxieties we have are often age-dependent; that is, they are related to our age and circumstances in life. Preschool-aged children have fairly predictable fears at various ages. Among two- to three-year-olds, for example, fears of animals, strangers, loud noises, unusual events, unexpected movements, and of course, Santa Claus, are common. By four to five years old, being afraid of the dark is also common.

Children can also develop phobias—fears that cause them to avoid normal activities or to shy away from commonly well-tolerated situations. For a seven-year-old to be afraid of a large, barking, and aggressive dog is reasonable and probably healthy. For a seven-year-old to be afraid of any dog, however small, friendly, and inoffensive, and to walk a block out of his way to avoid facing it even through a high, chain-link fence is phobic.

Parents often ask if they can transmit their own fears to their children, and the answer is a resounding yes! In our first few years of life, we form many of our initial likes and dislikes, food and color preferences, and a whole host of opinions about people and the world. Many of our opinions will stay with us our whole lives. Surrounded by the constant influence of their parents, children learn many of their preferences as if through osmosis. If we are phobic about swimming, for example, or heights, our anxiety is easily picked up by our children and is often internalized as their own. Mom and Dad are our primary models on how to view the world. It's small wonder that parents have such great influence on us.

Some children are more prone than others to develop anxieties. Sometimes they are simply more vulnerable to anxiety by nature and temperament; predisposition to certain types of fear, or even fearfulness itself, is probably heritable in some cases. Regardless of how our children develop fears and anxieties, however, with severe enough anxiety may come symptoms that may not be immediately associated with fear by the parent. Other signs of anxiety may be thumb-sucking, fingernail-biting, occasional incontinence, poor appetite, insomnia or hypersomnia, irritability, lethargy, and temper tantrums. Some parents will recognize that this list consists of behaviors and symptoms also classically associated with depression. And well it should: Anxious children often are also depressed.

Anxiety is an important symptom to recognize early, because undiagnosed and untreated anxieties may strongly interfere with a child's progress academically and socially. Those increased difficulties can generate greater future anxieties, and so on, putting the child in a downward spiral. Anxiety is treatable, and handled effectively, it need not interfere with your child's life. Ignored or untreated, specific anxieties, fears, or phobias often become generalized, causing problems in many areas of life. For instance, a child with a specific anxiety such as a fear of meeting or talking to new people, will begin to worry about the possibility of things going wrong in other areas, even when there is no obvious reason for their concern. They often worry about their performance in school, academically, athletically, and socially, even if they've not previously had problems in those areas.

Frequently, play therapy (see chapter ten) is used with great success to help the therapist identify the source of your child's anxiety, as well as to help your child resolve the issues that are the cause. Anxiolytic (antianxiety) medications are not needed for the treatment of anxiety in children as often as in adults. Your child's psychiatrist might choose no medication at all, or she might use one of several different antidepressants instead.

Although medication is often not necessary, a combination of play, talk, and family therapy might be.

Although professional help is sometimes needed with a very anxious child, parents can take some important steps on their own to help their children:

Reinforce self-esteem. Because anxious children are also depressed children, they often suffer low self-esteem. Taking the time to notice what children are doing and praising positive behavior, attitudes, and accomplishments goes far in helping children raise their self-esteem. Their increased self-esteem helps them to cope more effectively with their anxieties, in or out of therapy.

Although almost anything may be used to praise a child, it's important that whatever we praise is truly worthy of praise. Children have incredibly effective "baloney" detectors built in, and if you're being disingenuous, they'll know it. Your attempt to boost their self-esteem will not only *not* work, but it will also convince them even more of their lack of worth. They will feel even worse about themselves if they think that Mom and Dad feel so sorry for them that they are making up things to praise.

Reassure them of your love for them as a parent. Regardless of the source of your child's anxiety, reassurance of your love will help her. Frequent sources of anxiety include the child's misunderstanding of her worth, her abilities, liabilities, even imagined deformities. As a result, an anxious child often sees herself as unloved, sometimes as unlovable. Your frequent assurance of your belief in her, your regular affirmation of your continued love for her, your ongoing concern for her success, all combine to help the child improve her view of self.

Although some anxieties may make sense to you as a parent, others may not. More important to remember, whether the anxiety focus makes sense to you or not, is that your child is a child. His conceptualization of reality, of what's important, is not the same as an adult's. What *he* identifies as significant is the only reliable standard for determining how meaningful his concerns are to him. It's also important to remember that the child is not to blame for his anxiety. Even though the child's attitudes and understanding of the way the world works are primary to the establishment of his anxiety, having those attitudes and understanding is not a cause for blame. "Well, if you didn't have such silly thoughts about that, you would be fine!" is *not* an effective way to deal with a child who is anxious. Making the child see himself as "bad and wrong" for holding certain beliefs will cause him only more pain, more self-rejection, more anxiety. Helping the child to develop new ways of seeing the situation—ways that reduce his anxiety and concern—is far more likely to give him relief.

Situations that cause a change in daily routine need to be explained to the child within the context of his understanding. Particularly with a young child, events will occur that are so far removed from the normal daily routine that anxiety almost naturally results. The birth of a sibling, the arrival of an adopted child, a serious illness or death in the family, or a divorce all represent times when the most well-balanced child will undergo enormous stress. These situations will often create any of a number of anxieties in the child.

Unfortunately, many parents faced with these same circumstances are uncomfortable discussing them with their child. Sometimes these parents try to simply ignore the situation, hoping the child won't ask about it. Equally risky is the overcompensating parent who, nervous and distraught herself, overexplains, giving the child far more detail than he can possibly handle. This merely serves to increase the his anxiety. Recognizing your own discomfort with situations and discussing it with other adults before attempting to talk about it with your child is a far better course to follow. Understand that some things that happen will confuse, sadden, or frighten your child. He needs your adult interpretation and insight, but they must be tailored to *his* concerns and to *his* level of understanding, not yours. (See chapter seven for additional information on how to deal with these kinds of situation-specific anxieties in your child.)

Fears

As we've mentioned, parents can easily communicate their fears and phobias to their children, who often adopt them as their own. It's important first, then, to be aware of our own fears and concerns.

Understand that we are addressing what might be classified as unreasonable or excessive fears. All of us have some things or circumstances of which we are fearful. We might be afraid of cats, snakes, or bugs. We might be terrified of speaking in public, or driving in strange places; the list is endless. Although we may never have looked upon our own fears as excessive or unreasonable, taking a brief fear inventory of ourselves should reveal rather quickly those things or situations of which we are more fearful than most people. Keep in mind, too, that this is not an exercise in putting yourself down for having these fears and that this doesn't mean that we shouldn't or can't decide to take action to work on these fears.

Remember, though, that this is not the goal of the exercise. Instead, our goal is to recognize those things that make us unreasonably or excessively fearful, so we can avoid teaching our children to be fearful in the same way.

Even if we never let anything happen that might model our fears to our children, excessive fears will crop up in your child's life, if only because of the nature of how individuals become fearful. Usually, we become fearful by misunderstanding how a specific thing or occurrence relates to a negative or aversive circumstance in our life; we believe that the thing feared brings about the result to be avoided.

Even though excessive or unreasonable fears are almost impossible to avoid, when we realize that they exist, we need to help our children recognize the fallacy of their thinking. Particularly with a young child, the child's ability to see things in a realistic, logical light is limited. Here, supportive discussions with the child about his fear, showing understanding and concern, *not* belittling his fear, are called for. Disparaging a child for his fear will not help the child defeat the fear; it will simply convince the child that it isn't safe to discuss it with you!

Truly excessive fear, when it interferes with your child's functioning at home, school, or elsewhere, is a phobia. As hard as you might try to help your child with a phobia, it may well require professional help. Often you are too close to your child for the child to hear and believe you. Overcoming his fear might require behavioral or cognitive modification, which lends itself more to professional administration.

Fear can seem to be an exclusively negative emotion; but without fear, many of us would not live long enough even to have children! Of course, excessive fears and phobias are destructive. Realistic fears, however, are protective. They alert us to the presence of danger and give us the opportunity to recognize that danger and to proceed appropriately. Genuine danger needs to be recognized and avoided by your child. Although you want to alert your child to real dangers, you don't want her to become overly fearful or phobic. This can present a real dilemma. For example, you want your daughter to avoid getting into a car with a stranger, but you don't want to cause her to fear all strangers or to exacerbate her existing fear of strangers. Still, getting into a car with a stranger is a very real danger.

Real dangers must never be downplayed in an effort to avoid frightening a child unduly. You can present a warning to a child about a danger that he might encounter without causing unnecessary fear or diluting your concern. To be effective, discussions about dangers should be low key but presented in a serious fashion. A "family meeting" time is an excellent situation in which to discuss safety awareness with your child.

A family meeting is a regularly scheduled event. Families usually meet once a week on a preestablished day and time. The family meeting can be a pleasant affair but is not usually set up to be a fun time. Instead, it is set up with the children as a time to review recent events in the home, school, neighborhood, and community. It is not a complaint and grievance session for one child to express discontent about a sibling, nor is it a time set aside for the parent to complain about a child's behavior. Instead, it can be most effectively used as a time for the parents and the children to discuss how things are going in school, or, for example, how changes in a parent's or child's schedule affect the others, and it gives an opportunity for all to work on making changes that accommodate the family members.

During the family meeting, parents can discuss various topics over time. One evening, for example, you can consider dealing with strangers (for the younger children) and ways for the older children to comfortably refuse offers from peers to try a beer, a cigarette, or street drugs. By *discussing* these topics with the children rather than *lecturing* to them about your concerns, your interest in their safety seems less threatening, yet remains serious and important. Instead of frightening them with your concerns, you help them become partners in their own care. By discussing such situations with your children, you can often alleviate fears and anxieties.

The Shy Child

One of the most common fears in young children is that of meeting new people. Many young children are shy; they greet a newcomer while standing halfway behind Mom, a hint of a smile on their face. At the first hint of a sudden movement or a too-loud voice, they balk, hiding their face and their eyes in the back of Mom's leg. Over time, most children become more adventuresome and greet newcomers with great interest and without undue fear. But some children take much longer to achieve this level of confidence.

The child who is somewhat slow to warm to strangers may just be temperamentally more reserved than his more gregarious peers. If your child holds back when meeting other children, gentle encouragement to play with the newcomers may be enough to help him experiment with the social skills he has and to develop them further. Pushing a child to participate with others or showing anger at his shyness needs to be avoided, because it will only increase the child's anxiety. Sometimes it's enough to discuss your child's hesitance with him and to express your understanding. In other cases, the child may be able to identify those factors that cause him to be reluctant to associate with people new to him, opening the door to a productive discussion.

If your child's aversion to interacting with strangers seems mild and is not particularly troublesome, chances are good that your child is just temperamentally a little closer to the reserved end of the spectrum than to the highly social end. Although that child might always be a little more cautious about warming up to strangers, with time and greater experience, he will probably do well with strangers. But the child who shows an increasing lack of tolerance to situations where he meets and interacts with strangers or who demonstrates signs of terror and extreme anxiety is most likely a good candidate for intervention by a trained therapist.

The Angry and Aggressive Child

Anger and aggression are emotions that are developed normally within all human beings. Two of the most interesting facts noted in studying youngsters are the ease with which they can become angry and the amount of hostility that can develop within their aggressive expression.

Without the veneer of civility that comes with age and maturity, the bare aggression in some children that comes out of anger can be almost frightening in its intensity. Even so, it's important to remember that this aggression isn't abnormal, or even unusual, but merely representative of the child's immature emotional response to being frustrated, hurt, or thwarted in his aims. Even in adults, the sequence of emotional hurt, anger, then aggression is the most frequent response pattern among the emotionally unsophisticated. Interestingly, academic and intellectual achievement does not appear to modify this response; only those who have achieved emotional maturity seem able to respond with composure to hurt or frustration. Our children obviously don't possess this maturity; small wonder, then, that their anger can take such strong and aggressive forms.

Aggression: Innate, Learned, or Both?

Although it's true that some people have a genetic predisposition toward violent behavior and that that predisposition is sometimes passed on to their children, environmental factors seem just as important. Modeling of violent or aggressive behavior by parents, siblings, and friends, and watching violent acts on television have clearly been shown to increase the likelihood of a violent act by a child who is already predisposed to violence. This modeling of violent behavior may also increase the likelihood of a violent act by a characteristically nonviolent child.

Our society sends a confusing set of messages about violence to adults, let alone to children. Decrying violence generally, we seem to applaud violence perpetrated in the name of a "good cause": Successful military operations, even when they involve violence, death, and destruction, are an example. A heavy-handed police officer who strikes an intoxicated teenager in self-defense is often called abusive, but another officer who shoots and kills a robbery suspect may be termed a hero. If these different interpretations of violence are confusing to many adults, they are all the more so to our children.

Many families have grown to accept violence and aggression as a way of life, and children raised in this environment will come to adopt the family mores. In other families, aggression and violence are not acceptable, but they may not have demonstrated a firm and consistent alternative way of handling aggression to their children. One example of this inconsistency is the difference in the way some families deal with boys' and girls' aggression. For some, male children are expected to be more aggressive than girls. Aggression in girls is suppressed as "unladylike," whereas aggression in male children is often greeted with, "That's my boy!" Even though the parent realizes that the aggression is negative behavior, he almost approves of it, so he is less effective in dealing with the problems it may cause his child. At other times, the aggressive behavior is clearly unacceptable and is sanctioned heavily. This type of inconsistency in guidelines makes it more difficult for the child to learn to behave appropriately.

Abused children tend to be more violent and aggressive with peers than are children who have not been abused. Impulse control is often impaired in these children; their fantasies are often more violent, and they often are more hostile in general than children who have not been abused. As might be expected, children living in highly stressful home environments—where there is serious emotional discord among the parents, drug and alcohol abuse, physical or sexual abuse, serious financial problems, or frequent fights—are much more likely to show aggressive, even violent, behavior than children raised in homes without those stressors.

Dealing with Anger and Aggression

Coping with your child's anger and aggression is extremely stressful, particularly if you have no idea what's causing the behaviors. Without understanding the root of the anger (a physical assault, theft of a favorite toy, depression, et cetera), it's virtually impossible to help the child find an alternate expression. Even when the cause of the child's anger is known (by observation, discussion with the child, or the input of another child or adult), controlling the expression of aggression and rage remains paramount and may require intervention by a mental health professional.

Helping the child find alternatives to rage and hostility as methods of dealing with anger may prevent the progression to violence. Even when you isolate and deal with the reason for the anger, you still need to identify the model source. Where does your child learn his aggressive behaviors? In some cases, it's another child. If so, limit your child's exposure to that child. If that's not practical, make sure the children are supervised when together. If your child sees this behavior modeled in a day-care center, bring your concerns to the attention of the center's staff. Television, too, may be a source. Too often parents are relieved when their children are sitting quietly in front of the television, not realizing the violent behavior being observed. Without the maturity to recognize the violence for what it is—unconscionable acts against society or individuals—some children are drawn to the excitement, which is then reflected in their acting-out behaviors. Television, music, electronic video games, Internet access, et cetera, should always be supervised by an adult.

Consider your own behavior. Is it possible that your children are simply acting in accord with what they've learned from you and your spouse? Are there other significant adults (grandparents, aunts and uncles) living in the home who can be models for this behavior? Children may not easily see why aggression, rage, and violence are unacceptable. To make it easier for them to grasp, be consistent in how you deal with these behaviors. Punishing some acts but ignoring others confuses children. Using any type of corporal punishment for angry and aggressive behavior sends a mixed message to a child. Instead, remove privileges, such as favorite toys, television, or the use of the telephone, et cetera, for a specified period. Place the child in time-out. This gives the child the opportunity and safe space to regain control and prevents the escalation of angry feelings and actions. Teach other acceptable ways of dealing with anger and frustration, like punching a pillow or a punching bag, counting to ten, or writing down the feelings in a journal.

Preventing Aggression

As we've discussed, even children with a genetic predisposition to aggressive behavior become more aggressive after the behavior is modeled. Children without that tendency often learn the behaviors through such modeling.

Limiting aggressive and violent behavior often hinges on limiting your child's exposure to examples of such behavior. Preventing the child from witnessing televised violence and avoiding violence in your relationships at home will do much to prevent the development of aggressive and violent behavior in your child.

Most children have gained sufficient self-control by age three or four, and professional help usually is not indicated. However, in some cases, children will display such serious problems with aggression and violence toward other children, or even themselves (head-banging, cutting, biting), that outside help is needed. Severe, or continuous, aggressive acting-out behaviors by a young child or teen should always be called to the attention of a mental health professional. The longer the behavior is allowed to continue, the more difficult it becomes to break the destructive cycle.

PART III

Finding Help:
The Role of Therapy

NINE

A Parent's Role in a Child's Therapy

Because few parents consider it a minor step to call a social worker, psychologist, or child psychiatrist to evaluate their child, parents who do are already upset and stressed and probably have been for some time. Their child is upset, too, between problems at home with siblings, difficult if not hostile moments with Mom or Dad, and a whole series of problems at school.

What can parents do to support their child in therapy, be available for their child, and yet not interfere? How can they help in the therapeutic process?

Focus Your Energy

It may seem simple to discuss how important therapy may be for a child and how the parents can cooperate with the therapist and help with the goals of therapy, but when it's your child, it may seem overwhelming.

If you've decided that you're concerned enough about the behaviors you see in your child to consult a mental health professional, chances are good that you're feeling angry ("Why Johnny?"), fearful ("Can he be helped?"), confused ("Am I doing the right thing?"), along with a host of other emotions, most of them not at all helpful. Guilty feelings about what harm you may have done or whether you are inadequate or bad parents will probably beset you. Thoughts about what you've done wrong, what you could have done better or different, can assail you at every turn.

A key point in helping your child is to keep in mind that it's unlikely that you caused the problem. Although you try hard to be a good parent, no one is perfect. Being human means that you, too, have emotions. And being human, you may not always have made the best decisions or handled everything in the best possible fashion. Remember, too, that even among the "experts," few agree on everything. Occasionally (though not often) a parent may have done something so inappropriate as to cause or worsen their child's difficulties, but few parents, if any, are *entirely* responsible for their child's problems in life. Far more likely is that the child with long-term, serious difficulties may have a genetic predisposition that makes it easier for him to develop the symptoms he has. Sometimes, terrible events beyond the parents' control have contributed to the child's problems. However you may have contributed to your child's difficulties, you must also remember that right now you are the only one in a position to help your child. You must forgive yourself your imperfections and focus your emotional energy instead on helping your child.

Choosing a Therapist

In the appendices of this book is a list of national organizations that can provide more information about specific disorders and agencies that can refer you to a therapist in your area. The best referrals are professional referrals from people such as your family doctor, your child's pediatrician, the school psychologist or counselor, a professional organization, a local organization that deals with the specific needs of your child (CHADD groups for children with ADHD, for example), or your minister or rabbi. Using your resources to locate a therapist is more likely to lead to a competent one. However, if you are able to work only from a list of therapists assigned through your employer, clinic, or the court system, your choices are limited. Obviously the more therapists you have to choose from, the more likely you'll find one whose disposition and expertise are a match for you and your child.

Word of mouth can be very effective. Talk with as many people as you can about who is the best child psychiatrist, psychologist, or therapist in your area. Ask physicians, school teachers, anyone who works in a helping profession. Call different social service agencies. Get as many names from people as you can. Some names will keep popping up—those recurring names have a high chance of being good therapists for your son or daughter.

Referrals can also be obtained from your local medical society, mental health association or county mental health administrator, psychiatric society, or the American Academy of Child and Adolescent Psychiatry in Washington, DC.

Differences between Mental Health Professionals

There are differences between the various types of mental health professionals. We listed some of the differences here to give you a basic understanding of the many types of therapists available to work with children. No matter whom you eventually telephone for an appointment, be sure the therapist specializes in working with children and holds a license to practice in your state.

Psychiatrists are physicians (either M.D. or D.O.) who have earned a bachelor's degree and also either a medical degree or doctor of osteopathy degree. The undergraduate degree usually takes four years; both medical school and osteopathic medical school take an additional four years. Psychiatrists complete residency training that includes one year of internship. To be eligible to be board certified in general psychiatry, a four-year residency is required. For child and adolescent psychiatry, a three-year residency in general psychiatry is needed, plus two additional years in a child and adolescent psychiatry fellowship.

Psychiatrists are trained in both psychotherapy and the use of psychopharmacological agents; they are the only mental health professionals who can write prescriptions. Trained first as physicians, they are aware of important mind-body interactions and are able to determine if seemingly psychological symptoms are actually caused by a physical illness. Their expertise in the use of psychopharmacological agents will be required if medications are needed, regardless of the type of mental health professional you use.

Although not all emotional or psychological difficulties (mental illnesses) will require the use of medications, many do. In general, the more serious the illness, the greater the likelihood that medication will be part of the therapeutic regimen. In the event that you choose a nonpsychiatrist mental health professional and medications are required, the other professional will refer you to a psychiatrist she is familiar with and trusts.

Psychologists are mental health professionals who have earned either a Ph.D. (doctor of philosophy) in clinical psychology or a Psy.D. (doctor of psychology). In addition to a bachelor's degree, they have generally studied at least three additional years at the graduate level in psychology, with emphasis on personality theory, psychotherapy, and psychodynamics. Their training also includes a great deal of supervised clinical work. Requirements for licensure vary from state to state but will likely include at least one year of such work, usually more.

In addition to providing psychotherapy, clinical psychologists provide psychological testing, either for their own use with clients or for other mental health professionals. Fully licensed to practice independently, psychologists often work together with psychiatrists. In those cases, the psychologist usually provides psychological testing and psychotherapy, and the psychiatrist prescribes needed medications as well as coordinates any necessary medical care.

Social workers have taken a position of increasing importance as providers of mental health services in recent years. Those with special training and expertise in evaluating and treating emotional and psychiatric difficulties are called clinical or psychiatric social workers. They usually hold a master's degree in social work (M.S.W. or M.S. in social work) and are licensed by the state they work in.

Even more so than psychologists, most social workers are associated with psychiatrists, working closely with them to help resolve their clients' difficulties. In many smaller communities, social workers are the only mental health professionals available, and the services they provide are of great importance.

Psychiatric nurse practitioners have completed general nurse training, most often at the bachelor of science level, then continued through the master's level in nursing, with specialized training in mental health. They receive supervised training in the treatment of mental illness, often practicing independently, especially in those states that have legisled insurance reimbursement for their services.

Although they are not physicians, they have training that gives them insight to the medical aspects of psychiatric illness. As with the nonmedical mental health professionals, they are often associated with psychiatrists; many have office space and work alongside psychiatrists in their offices.

Mental health counselor is a term that has been unregulated and unlicensed until recently. In slightly fewer than half of the fifty states the term is still undefined and unregulated. In the other states a new professional degree has developed. Awarded after a two-year master's program has been completed, it includes specialized study in counseling as well as supervised clinical work and is often referred to as an M.C., or master's in counseling. Although qualified to provide psychotherapy and entitled to the term *psychotherapist*, most M.C.s prefer to call themselves counselors.

Marriage and family therapists are not considered a specific specialty in most states; professionals who specialize in this area usually identify themselves first by their main professional identification, adding that they specialize in marriage and family therapy—for example, a psychiatric social worker specializing in marriage and family therapy.

Their numbers will probably increase as demand increases for this type of specialization; currently approximately twenty states license marriage and family therapists. California has a license category of MFCC, or marriage, family and child counselor.

Although small in number, as this profession matures, marriage and family counselors will take on an increasingly important role. Even now, particularly well-qualified marriage and family counselors provide important services to their clients.

Calling for an Appointment

Unless you are calling a major medical center, a social service agency, or a therapist in a large practice, your phone call may be answered by an answering machine. If this happens, just leave your name and phone number and the best time to reach you. There is no reason to leave a message on the machine or with a secretary or receptionist as to why you are calling other than to say you would like to set up an appointment for your child. Rarely when you telephone will you be able to speak with the therapist. She will return your call and set up an appointment with you. Be wary of a receptionist who asks the specific reason for your call. This is confidential information that is reserved for the therapist.

Fees

Fees for therapy depend on the education and credentials of the therapist, the therapy setting, and your locale. In major metropolitan areas the fee for services is usually higher than that in rural areas. Also, fees for services provided in a clinic setting will be lower than fees in a private practice.

Before beginning therapy, parents should check their health insurance policy to see how much is allocated for mental health services. This information can also be obtained directly from your employer, or, as is often the case nowadays, the therapist's office staff can make an inquiry for you directly to the insurance provider—they will need your insurance card, so be sure to bring it with you if you want them to make the inquiry for you.

If you do not have insurance, some therapists have a fee schedule that permits families to pay "based on their income" or their "ability to pay." The fee is lower than it would be for someone whose income is higher or for someone who carries insurance. Usually treatment that is based on your ability to pay will be available in a clinic setting or at a social service agency.

Children under the age of eighteen who are U.S. citizens or legal aliens and are blind or disabled are eligible for Supplemental Security Insurance (SSI) payment if the family income is low. Call your local Social Security office to determine what the income limits are or obtain additional information from the Social Security Administration at (800) 772-1213. Anyone who is eligible for SSI will also be eligible for Medicaid, a health insurance program usually run by the state's social service department.

Preparing for Your First Meeting

A small amount of preparation before you first meet the therapist you are considering will help make that visit far more effective. Remember, this is a preliminary consultation. Nothing should be chiseled in stone. Unless you've used this person before or know him personally, you might prefer to wait until after this first meeting to decide whether you'll be comfortable using his services. Regardless of how well recommended to you he comes, as a parent you must be comfortable dealing with him. You and the therapist will become partners in helping your child. Don't sign on as a partner until you meet him and have discussed your child with him. After all, your child's therapist is the one to whom you'll be looking for guidance and help in making important decisions about your child. This is the person to whose judgment you might well be entrusting your child's welfare.

Preparing for your first meeting will take a little time, but it will be time well spent. Parents who have copies of medical reports, school records, occupational or physical therapy reports, or results of psychological evaluations should be prepared to bring these documents to the initial appointment. These records can usually save a great deal of time and assist with the evaluation.

If you are able to provide a list of symptoms that will help the therapist understand your child better, do so. Little things that you have noticed about your child are sometimes very important to the therapist. For instance, if your child tends to have little eye contact with others, flaps his arms, takes things apart constantly, has obsessive thoughts or compulsive acts, or never understands a joke, these are important observations to bring into the first meeting. Too often, we tend to list complaints ("Last week was awful, and I thought I would lose my mind") rather than address the real issues that concern us. Be specific and resist the urge to ramble on about the latest episode in full detail during the consultation meeting.

Part of preparation means taking out a piece of paper and writing out a number of things about your child that you probably haven't reviewed for a while. You'll want to ask yourself some questions as you sit and think about who your child is and how to describe her.

Pregnancy

Even if your child is a teen, there are things about his early life that the therapist will be interested in. Go back to the beginning. Take notes as you recollect, so that you will find it easier to document later. Was the mother's pregnancy normal and uneventful, or did she have any medical problems or accidents? During the pregnancy, did your child need or receive any medical care in utero? Even if the pregnancy and delivery were relatively normal, did the mother have any serious medical conditions through her pregnancy, even if they started before she was pregnant? Consider heart, liver, and kidney ailments as serious. Did she have diabetes prior to pregnancy, or did she develop diabetes while pregnant? Now, think of his birth. Was it easy and uncomplicated, or was his mother in labor for many hours? Was he a breech baby? Were forceps used? Was he delivered by Cesarean section? Was he premature, or was he long overdue? Was labor induced?

Did he have any medical problems while in the hospital before going home? Newborns usually go home within a day or two after birth, three at the most. If there were no complications, how long was he in the hospital before being sent home?

First Year

The first year of life is important in terms of a child's later development. Did she seem to develop normally and along a similar timeline as other infants you've known, or were you aware of significant delays? Did she go to the doctor for regular well-baby checks, and if she did, were her checkups always normal? How old was she when she first sat up unaided, when she spoke her first words? At what age did she start to crawl? When could she stand while holding on to something, and when could she stand unaided? When did she take her first step? Though it might seem like a lot of information, it's important for the person evaluating your child—unless it's impossible to provide because the child was adopted. If your child's baby book is available, take that with you to the appointment.

Medical Problems

Make a note of any unusual medical problems your child has had as he's grown up. Include the usual childhood diseases only if he had a particularly tough time with any of them. List any current medical problems. If he's taking medication, list the names of those prescriptions, the dosages, and the number of times per day he takes the medication. Also include any over-the-counter medications that the child takes regularly.

School

No matter the age of the child, if he's attended school, spend some time thinking about his school performance. Has he generally done well in school, or has school been difficult? Has he had behavioral problems in school, just academic difficulties, both, or neither? Have teachers made any specific comments about his ability to learn, to behave, to attend (pay attention effectively)? Whether you acted on it or not, did anyone at school (educator, nurse, counselor) ever share concerns about possible difficulties in learning or behaving? Has your child frequently been in trouble in school, and if so, what kind of trouble? How have his grades been?

The Child as a Whole Person

Now let's start to think about your child as the whole person that she is. Start with her appearance. Does she usually look neat and clean, or does she seem to have a cloud of dust following her, even right after she gets out of the bath? Is she concerned with her appearance, or would she walk around in the same unwashed clothes for a week if you'd let her? Think a bit about her room and her play areas. Some children seem to be neat and orderly from the moment of birth; some never are. Some children are neat, but almost compulsively so; for these children, any little thing out of place can send them into a panic. Is your child neat, a little too neat for you to be comfortable, or unbothered by clutter altogether?

How would you describe your child's personality? Some children are gregarious and active, will speak with anyone, and do anything that occurs to them. Other children are fairly active, friendly, even outgoing, but somewhat more reserved than the former group. Some children are strictly loners, staying in their room, or at least close to home. Some children follow easily, some children prefer to lead; some choose to do neither, spending most of their time in solitary pursuits. There are children who can be described only as bright and sunny; their disposition could melt snow! But there are also children who would be described as dark and cloudy. Most children are somewhere in the middle.

Last, consider what your thoughts are about your child today. What would you say about his problems? Is there one big problem or a group of smaller but important problems? Are you most concerned about his attitudes, or do his behaviors worry you more? What does his mental state seem like to you? Do you think he's depressed? If you do think he's depressed, what's your evidence? If not, why not? Be thoughtful here; remember that children often express depression differently than adults do. In fact, they often express a number of emotions differently than adults do. Review the chapters in the second section of this book to be alert to the kinds of symptoms children can display that might indicate problems with depression, anxiety, or other mental and emotional difficulties.

Whether you realize it or not, a parent plays an important role in a partnership with the therapist. The parent is privy to information about the child that only he can relate to the therapist. Even the child is incapable of relaying this type of information about himself. Taking the time to think about and sort through your feelings and observations about your child will be of great assistance to a therapist—and ultimately a benefit to your child.

Your First Meeting with the Therapist

When you first meet with the person who will evaluate your child, answer her questions honestly. Help her to understand your child and his behavior as honestly as you can.

Many times, psychological and other tests may be ordered for your child, but the most time-honored and frequently the most valuable element of understanding your child and his problem is history. Certain disorders or problems have a distinct natural history of how they start and progress, so the more specific you are in answering questions, the more complete and rapid the therapist's understanding of your child is likely to be.

Most therapists will want to see or test your child over more than one visit before making a diagnosis. Often, the therapist will also want to meet with you more than once before making a diagnosis. A complete evaluation can be detailed and lengthy and is not inexpensive, so help the evaluator do the best job she can. An incorrect evaluation and diagnosis can steer your child and his therapist in the wrong direction, wasting time and money and delaying effective treatment.

Talking to the evaluator or the evaluation team is important, but so is listening to them. Ask them questions that will help you understand the process and give you a sense of participation. When you're given an answer, quite often you'll be asked if you understand. If you don't, don't let embarrassment or the fear of looking silly or unintelligent force you to say you understand when you don't! To most parents, few things in life are as important as the welfare of their children. Not understanding the jargon or concepts used should not become a source of shame. Ask your questions, repeat the answers in your own words, and determine if you truly understand. If you do—great! If you don't, have the therapist explain in a different way.

At the end of the first session, the therapist and you will agree to a schedule for regular appointments. It's important for you and your child that the schedule stay the same for the duration of the therapy if the treatment is to succeed. Sessions normally last from forty-five to fifty minutes. If you are late, don't expect the session to run over the normal time because it is important to other patients that they be seen on time. If, however, the therapist is running late, then it is reasonable to expect that you will receive a full session.

Before the Conclusion of the First Meeting
Any specific questions you have about the therapist and his plans should be asked before you leave the first meeting. These may include the following:

• What are his fees?

• How you can reach her if there's an emergency?

• Who takes his calls if he's away from the office?

• What is her specialty (NBDs, depression, ADD/ADHD, LDs)?

• How long has she been treating children like yours?

• Does he use medication (if not, and your child needs medication, to whom does he refer you)?

• Does she work with the school if your child is having academic problems?

• How long does he estimate therapy might last?

• What type of treatment does she think will help your child?

• Are parents involved in the treatment?

Lastly, ask the therapist how he usually maintains communication with parents. The laws of confidentiality protect children and adults, but the laws do not protect children from parents. Some therapists will tell you everything, whereas other therapists will not tell you anything. But many therapists take the middle road; they share but do not give you the particulars. There are limitations on these laws, but they vary from state to state. If your child is an adolescent, little if any information will be shared. However, at all ages, should your child threaten suicide or other bodily harm, threaten to hurt another person, or threaten to destroy property, the therapist will share this information with you.

A therapist rarely, if ever, discusses a patient with a spouse or employer. Yet, psychosocial interventions with a child usually involve not only the child, but also his parents, and also the school to an extent. This exchange of information is needed for the child to receive dynamically oriented therapy along with medication and special educational services.

Other people, like the child's pediatrician, may know that the child is in therapy, but the pediatrician has no right to know what the child tells the therapist. Sharing treatment plans and goals of therapy is not the same as sharing confidential information with the pediatrician in the case of a child.

Parents who are divorced have equal access to the child's therapist if they are both custodial parents. However, in the case of single custody the noncustodial parent must obtain permission from the custodial parent to be involved in the treatment of the child.

After the First Appointment

When you walk out of the first meeting with the therapist, you should feel relieved—relieved that you have found someone to help you with your child's problems. You should feel confident that the therapist knows what he is talking about and that it is possible to have a working partner relationship with him. Any questions you had should have been answered, if possible. You should feel confident that you'll have the right to ask for progress reports and that you can telephone if you have a question and need an answer quickly. But most of all, you should feel comfortable with the therapist. If you don't feel confident that this person will be able to help your child, then look for another therapist. If the therapist seemed to blame you for the child's problems, look for another therapist. Trust your instincts.

As many parents who have children in therapy can tell you, finding the right therapist for your child is sometimes difficult. Often parents who have a child with several diagnoses are very knowledgeable themselves. Sometimes a therapist is threatened by the parents' knowledge of the child's disorder or disorders, whereas another therapist may feel that her burden is a little lighter because of the parents' knowledge. Again, follow your instincts.

After the Diagnosis

After the diagnosis is made, you should meet again with the therapist. During this session, the therapist can explain what the diagnosis means and how it was made. She can also tell you what her immediate plans are for treatment. Two concepts are important here: the treatment plan and the goals of therapy.

The therapist will tell you what the treatment plan is; if this information is not volunteered, ask. The treatment plan is similar in essence to the game plan in a football game. It lays out how the therapy will begin, how it will progress, and the intermediate steps that need to be achieved before advancing. It will include the type of therapy that is planned and the steps it will involve.

The goals of therapy are related to the treatment plan but different. When the therapy is started, what the therapist hopes to achieve and roughly when she hopes to achieve it can be stated as the goals of therapy. Simply asked, what does the therapist hope to achieve through therapy? If the child is aggressive, hostile, and defiant, is therapy aimed at reducing that aggression and hostility and helping the child be more compliant? If the child lies and steals, is the goal of therapy to help the child stop lying and stealing?

Lastly, between the treatment plan and the goals of therapy, what will be the indices of success? That is, how will the therapist (and you, the parent) know that the child has achieved the goals of therapy, that the treatment plan has been effective? Your child's therapist should be willing to discuss these issues with you and to tell you what she thinks. Considering the important responsibility you're giving her—helping you to help your child—it is important that you understand how she will proceed and why.

Homework

You've heard the diagnosis and how it was reached. You've gone over the treatment plan and the goals of therapy, and you're comfortable that you and your child should proceed. What now? Discuss with the therapist your role in the therapy—how he plans for you to assist in the therapeutic process and what your "homework" will be.

Often, the therapist will ask you to keep track of the target behaviors or target symptoms. He may want to know how often they are occurring, how the child responds to your correction, and generally how and when you're seeing an improvement—or worsening—in the child's behavior overall. Though it may sound ominous, some children may actually have a short period of worsening of symptoms as they start therapy. Some children are fearful that they may be "changed" by therapy in a way they won't like. Others are resistant to giving up control of their behavior to the therapist. Regardless of these and other causes, seeing an initial worsening of symptoms at the start of therapy is neither rare nor, usually, of great concern.

The therapist will also probably appreciate reports of how the child is relating to other family members as well as his behavior and performance in school. Some therapists will rely on you for those school reports; others will ask permission to request reports directly from the teacher involved. Both methods are acceptable.

Your child's therapist may also want you to initiate some plan for behavioral change. It might be a token economy system, in which the child, in return for accomplishing certain activities (such as doing homework without being reminded or getting ready for bed when first asked with no argument), is given tokens that can be redeemed for certain privileges later. This token economy system might consist simply of keeping score on a tally sheet where the child can see the positive marks he has earned through the day. Preagreed levels of positive marks may be exchanged for privileges, similar to the use of tokens. There are numerous systems for tracking and modifying behavior, some simple, some more sophisticated. If your child's therapist recommends that you use one, be sure you understand its proper use.

It's possible that the therapist will also recommend other activities with your child, such as going together to the library, going for walks during which you can discuss your child's progress, reading with your child, et cetera. These types of activities can often be quite helpful, so be open to them.

Depending on the type of problems your child is experiencing, therapy may be relatively brief, or it might be lengthy. Either way, don't expect a miracle cure. Some children move forward faster than others. Some problems lend themselves to quicker resolution or improvement than others. Very few children will show tremendous improvement immediately.

Depending on your child and on the types of problems he's experiencing, you should see progress over time. To help assure yourself that things are progressing satisfactorily, as well as to stay effectively involved in your child's therapy, it's important at the start of therapy that you establish with the therapist scheduled meetings. These may be very brief and on the telephone or in person. Often, the therapist will want to meet with you for a few minutes before or toward the end of your child's session, either every visit or every other visit. This gives both you and the therapist an opportunity to discuss new developments and to share concerns and progress.

Parentwork

If you think that what was just discussed is parentwork, you're right. But there's more to parentwork than what we've talked about. During the course of your child's therapy, it's likely that your child's therapist will want to have some sessions with you. These meetings will be to discuss with you in detail how the therapy is going. More specifically, the therapist will discuss with you what he or she has found that you can work on with your child.

In these sessions the therapist can suggest how you can best help your child. Perhaps Johnny wants to do everything after school, but then becomes overwhelmed by the social commitments he's made. The therapist might ask you to help Johnny with prioritizing his activities, so that he can do what he most wants to do without overloading himself. Megan, on the other hand, may have hit a slump in her studies. Because she is just twelve years old, you might not anticipate that hormonal changes are affecting her concentration; gentle questioning, however, reveals that her breasts are often sore and that their sudden growth has captured much of her attention. Spending time with her, discussing what these changes mean, may make a positive change in your relationship as well as return her schoolwork to the "A" level it's always been. Helping you to help your child should be an important priority for the therapist.

Ghosts in the Nursery

A crucial part of parentwork has to do with what have been called "ghosts in the nursery." This refers to the feelings and experiences of your own childhood becoming superimposed on your child's life, as if part of your early life is relived through your child.

More clearly, it means that how you parent your child is likely to reflect your own childhood experiences, good and bad. In a larger sense, it can refer to the fact that our personality structures, for better or worse, will strongly influence how we parent our children. These last two facts will concern the therapist the most.

The bulk of our discussion on working with the therapist has focused on just that—working with the therapist in ways that help the child directly. Here the focus is on you, the parent, as an individual with your own life, your own history, your own difficulties in life. The focus is also on the fact that you have the primary responsibility for raising this child effectively. Keep in mind that the therapist's primary concern is your child. He will not be psychoanalyzing you or looking for ways to blame you for your child's problems.

What he will do is help you see possible blind spots, if they exist, that might be interfering with your ability to most effectively parent your child. You may, for example, have had demanding and perfectionistic parents. As a child, you might have been held to standards that exceeded any reasonable expectation of achievement. Your parents' unreasonable demands on your performance might have been crushing; no matter how well you did, it was never good enough.

When children grow up they often forget the lessons of their own childhood and, in fact, are likely to inflict on their own children what was inflicted on them—intentions to the contrary notwithstanding. In situations like these, your child's therapist will attempt to help you make some changes in your outlook that could help you achieve even more effective parenting skills. Your child's therapist is not there to criticize or evaluate you and should do neither. Nor will he attempt therapy with you. He will merely point out ways you can become an even better parent to your child. This will be further discussed in chapter eleven.

Working with a child means working with that child's family, at least with the parents, to help them help their child. Sometimes the therapist may believe that family therapy is in order and will recommend it. Understand that a recommendation for family therapy is not a criticism of you or your family. Remember that your child's behavior and attitudes develop not in a vacuum but rather in the context of her family. Your child's therapist believes that your child's progress and prognosis will improve greatly if members of your family are helped to relate to each other more effectively.

It's been shown that parents are more likely to be critical of their children or to become overinvolved when they are confused or lack knowledge of the problem or disorder. Without basic knowledge, parents often will ascribe the problem behavior to factors that are actually under the child's control. Parents need education, support, and a social network with other families whose children have the same diagnosis. As well, they often must learn effective coping skills because children with emotional, behavioral, and learning disorders can be challenging to parents. The stress of living with a child who has challenging behaviors branches off to all members of the family—no one in the family is spared.

Monitoring the Treatment

We've outlined the basic way a therapist should work with you and your child. The most significant parts of therapy that a parent must know are the treatment plan and the goals of therapy. After a therapist is able to provide you with a diagnosis, it is imperative that the treatment plan and the goals of therapy be outlined for you. If they are not, find out why. You have a right to this information.

Too often parents complain that their child has been in therapy for months, even years, and they have no idea what the therapist is trying to accomplish. A therapist who cannot tell you what his goals for therapy include is a red flag. If he cannot tell you what his goals are, how will he know when he has reached them?

Most therapists who specialize in working with children are conscientious, effective, and genuinely concerned about helping your child grow and improve. But what if you've seen no substantial improvement in attitude or behavior over a long period of time? What is a "long period of time" when speaking about a child in therapy? If you have doubts about whether your child's therapist is effective, what can you do?

Although you probably don't want to be confrontational, if you have these kinds of questions, a separate meeting with the therapist is in order. You child will soon notice your lack of enthusiasm for his treatment and his therapist if the doubts you harbor are not resolved, so discussing your doubts in a separate meeting with the therapist is in everyone's best interest.

Unfortunately, there are no hard and fast rules to determine whether your child's therapy is progressing effectively. Aside from the possible slight worsening of symptoms at the initiation of therapy, improvement should be noted over time, even if it is occasionally uneven. An appropriate timeframe is difficult to generalize, because the nature and severity of your child's illness figure prominently in determining how rapidly he can be expected to move noticeably forward. If several months go by without any improvement in attitude or behavior that you can see, discuss this with the therapist. There may be good reasons for this apparent plateau that she can explain to you. If you notice your child having trouble maintaining the status quo or actually worsening over time, it is appropriate to voice your concern to the therapist immediately.

In the worst case, you may ultimately come to believe that, for whatever reason, this therapist is not being effective with your child. Not every therapist is a good "fit" with every client or patient; even highly qualified therapists probably do better with some children than with others. Rather than wait, hoping for a change, consult your primary physician or the professional who referred you initially and let her know how you feel. Although it's important not to change therapists unnecessarily, continuing your child in therapy that is proving unsuccessful is worse than "unhelpful." It may actually be making your child's problems more difficult to deal with effectively.

Almost as troublesome as staying too long with an ineffective therapist is giving up too soon on one who truly is effective with your child. How could that happen? More easily than it would seem. The nature of the illness can help make some children resistant to therapy; the more they seem to improve, the more it seems that they compensate for their improvement in one area by worsening in another. If you notice this pattern developing as your child's therapy progresses, don't hesitate to discuss it with the therapist. Unfortunately, studies have shown that a great number of people leave therapy not when *they* are ready, but rather when their mental health insurance benefits run out.

Obtaining good therapy for your child is usually not that difficult; there are many excellent therapists in the field. However, as the following story will demonstrate, some children have myriad symptoms, sometimes making the actual diagnosis difficult to establish.

Tony, at age four, was diagnosed with attention deficit hyperactivity disorder. He began weekly therapy and a regimen of Ritalin (a stimulant medication used for treating children with ADHD) and did quite well for a few years. But during those years Tony's mother, Ann, began to notice other behaviors that disturbed her—some obsessive thoughts, difficulty making friends, and inappropriate behaviors in school and in the home. When Ann's father was diagnosed with cancer, Tony, then eight, showed absolutely no empathy. It was as if he was in his own world, unaware of how sick his grandfather was.

When Tony was nine, Ann became concerned because he was spitting, clapping his hands, and obsessing about germs. She mentioned her concerns to Tony's psychiatrist—the second psychiatrist Tony had seen through the years. The doctor and she both decided to watch Tony more closely. Weeks later the repetitive behaviors were worse, but Tony continued to deny to the doctor that he could not control the movements—even though he had told Ann that the spitting and hand-clapping could not be controlled.

A year later, Tony was plagued by repetitive thoughts and motions and had begun missing school because of this. However, Tony continued to deny that he couldn't control himself, and the psychiatrist refused to place him on medication until Tony admitted he had a problem. After much reading and talking with members of her support group, Ann began to believe that Tony had not only ADHD, but also obsessive-compulsive disorder—or at least symptoms of the disorder.

One day Tony told Ann that he "just can't tell him [the therapist] about it." She attempted one more time to talk with the therapist, but the conversation hit a dead end. It was then that Ann decided to seek a second medical opinion.

Meeting with a new psychiatrist, Ann recounted Tony's medical history. The doctor, concerned, asked Ann to set up an appointment so he could meet Tony. In the meantime, the new psychiatrist said he would review all of Tony's medical records.

At the next visit, the psychiatrist met with Tony privately. During Tony's second visit, he gave Tony, now eleven years old, a questionnaire to complete. Afterward he asked Ann to come into his office. There he told her that Tony was displaying many symptoms of obsessive-compulsive disorder—so many, in fact, that he was diagnosing him with the disorder. Ann found herself breathing a sigh of relief. Finally, she thought, Tony will be treated for a disorder that has plagued him for years!

The new psychiatrist explained to Ann what obsessive-compulsive disorder is and what he would be doing to help Tony. But he also told her that he still had some concerns about Tony and that he would be observing Tony carefully over the next few sessions.

A month later, after Tony had been seeing the new doctor weekly, the doctor requested a private meeting with Ann. It was at this meeting that Ann learned that Tony also displayed characteristics of Asperger's disorder (see chapter four). The doctor told Ann about Asperger's and then advised that she read and learn more about it, and he recommended a list of book titles to her. He then shared his treatment plan and goals of therapy with Ann and told her what she could do to help Tony at home.

In this story, we first see that there was a poor fit between the second therapist and the child—the child refused to talk to the therapist about his compulsive thoughts and obsessive actions. Even Mom was having difficulty communicating with the doctor. It was apparent to Mom that after twenty months of therapy, her son was not being helped. Mom's intuition also told her that something else was going on with her son, that what she was observing wasn't *just* ADHD. And she was right. The saddest part of this story, of course, is that Tony went untreated for so many years, preventing him from experiencing a relatively normal childhood and development.

Unfortunately, situations like this do develop, albeit not often, but it confirms that parents are still their child's best advocate. It's important that parents continue to rely on their intuition. If something doesn't feel right, if your questions and concerns are not taken seriously and addressed appropriately, it's time to move on to another therapist. If your child isn't improving, and you're suspicious that the diagnosis isn't accurate, it's worth traveling to a university, medical center, or hospital that has a child and adolescent psychiatric division to obtain a diagnosis from top professionals in the field.

Your child's therapy can open doors to his life and future that were previously closed and locked. It can stop or reduce pain that your child is experiencing now, as well as prevent a great deal of pain in the future. Although not a magic wand, therapy can often offer possibilities not otherwise imaginable. You may find, however, as other parents have, that your child isn't the only one who will grow with his therapy!

TEN

Understanding the Types of Therapy

You started out concerned about your child, and so you're reading this book looking for answers. You've learned a great deal about what you can expect from a good therapist. You're better prepared to be effective in working with him from the first consultation. You understand better than before what an effective therapist can help your child achieve.

You've learned that this is not a "parent-passive" operation. Our personal experience tells us that you've probably already learned far more than you ever intended to or wanted to about what may be happening within your child, but you also know more about the people you can turn to for help. If you are having a difficult time with your child now, you can also appreciate the enormous burden she feels, as well. You may at times have been angry at your child or embarrassed by her behavior or attitudes. You may have wondered why these difficulties had been visited upon you. But as you continue to read, we believe you will continue to grow in your commitment to help your child improve the quality of her life today and her life tomorrow.

The therapist you choose will work hard to help your child, and you will, too. You probably weren't prepared to hear just how much effort might be required on your part, but you're strong—you'll stand your ground.

If your child has more than the "garden variety" growing pains, you may have some difficult days ahead of you. Now it's time to learn about what may be happening inside your child and what can be done to help him. The more prepared you are to understand how and why he is as he is, the more effective you can be in working with your child and the therapist to help your child accomplish the most he can. The worst days will end, but

178

they may still be before you. Learn what is possible and what will work best for your family and your child.

In this chapter, we'll present "snapshot views" of the therapeutic options you're most likely to have available to you. Keep in mind that the number of choices you'll have will depend, to a large degree, on where you live. If you're in a large city located almost anywhere in this country, your choices should be as varied as the therapies we'll present here. If you live in a more rural area, practical issues will probably limit you to fewer choices.

But more is not always better. It's been our experience as well as that of our professional associates that some therapies work better than others for certain types of emotional difficulties. But we've also found that it's the artist, not the instrument, who makes the music. And so it is with therapists and therapy. A therapy that's rationally based and organized along clearly validated, scientifically demonstrated principles will always do better than a "by guess and by golly" approach thrown together by someone who sees the new and sensational as profitable.

But it's also a fact that the most sophisticated therapies will never accomplish what they are capable of when administered by the ill-prepared. What has proven consistently true over time is that the well-prepared and well-followed proven technique can accomplish what must be done to help others as much as they can be helped.

So if you live in a place where everything from psychoanalysis to tea-leaf reading is available, consider yourself lucky. If not, don't feel cheated. The latest and greatest is often just the latest— not the greatest. A competent, caring therapist who enjoys working with troubled young people, helping them to grow and learn, can be as effective in your part of the country as anywhere else, whether you live on Park Avenue or Main Street, USA.

The therapies that are discussed next are among those most widely—and successfully—used today. The list is not exhaustive; new ideas and trends develop almost daily. But a good therapist who will work with you and your child using any of these therapies—and some that, inevitably, we won't have mentioned—can be immensely helpful to your child, and the work that you will accomplish together may bear fruit for years to come.

In the past twenty years, psychological and psychiatric therapy has seen a veritable explosion in the number and types of therapy promoted and practiced. Most mainstream mental health professionals who work largely or exclusively with children, however, use a comparative "handful" of therapeutic perspectives and techniques. New techniques are being developed all the time, so it's important that the mental health professional you choose stays up to date. It's equally important, however, that your therapist not be given to investing your time and money exploring new and unproven therapies. What follows is a list of broad classifications of the most frequently used therapeutic techniques.

Psychodynamic Therapies

Psychoanalytic theory, closely associated by most people with Sigmund Freud, provided us with the concepts that define psychodynamics. Psychoanalysis, a long (three to five years average), intense (three to five sessions per week), and obviously expensive proposition, is unwieldy. Its use in child and adolescent therapy has largely fallen from favor, primarily because of its cost and extreme length.

Since psychoanalysis was first proposed as a treatment modality, however, psychoanalytic principles have been refined and clarified, and that body of data forms the basis for psychodynamic therapies. Most simply put, psychodynamics is the study of how the unconscious mind interacts with the conscious mind and of how unresolved conflicts in the unconscious affect one's conscious thought, outward behavior, and manner of coping with life.

Psychodynamic therapists believe that *insight* regarding these conflicts, brought to the light of conscious thought, helps the patient resolve these conflicts in a way that promotes his greater mental health and enjoyment of life. As in psychoanalysis, *interpretation* of the patient's thoughts and behavioral styles gives the therapist insight into the patient's unresolved unconscious conflicts. These interpretations are then shared with the patient at a pace and in a manner the patient can tolerate; he is given the time and given the help necessary to work through his problem areas.

Even in situations in which sharing the interpretations with the patient or client wouldn't be of much help to her because of a child's lack of emotional and intellectual maturity, for instance, the understanding of psychodynamic principles by the therapist is still of enormous value to the therapy. The therapist can still guide the individual's therapy to help her make the important connections at an unconscious level, even if those connections would be too arcane or too complex for the child to deal with effectively at a conscious level. Improvement can still occur.

Most of the other forms of therapy rely, to a greater or lesser extent, on the therapist's understanding and ability to apply psychodynamic concepts with his patients or clients. Often, psychodynamic therapy is combined effectively with many other types of therapy, notably with biological therapy (see following), in which the use of medications is combined with psychodynamic talk therapy.

Look at the following situation for an example of how a child who might be too emotionally and intellectually immature to deal with a psychodynamic interpretation can still benefit greatly from the *therapist's* understanding.

Until the birth of his sister, Sarah, two months ago, Marshall was a typical, energetic, inquisitive, and basically happy three-year-old. At thirty-nine months, his physical, emotional, and intellectual maturity is actually at the high end of normal. But since the arrival of Sarah, he's had trouble sleeping. Totally day and night toilet-trained for two months before Sarah came home, he's had occasional accidents, usually wetting at night, with some wetting and soiling during the day.

A friendly, outgoing, happy, and compliant child in the past, he's become almost isolative at times; but when Mother tends to feeding, changing, or bathing Sarah, Marshall interrupts Mother, demands her attention, yells, and throws toys at her and the walls. In the last two weeks, Mrs. Nelson, Marshall's mother, has caught him several times standing quietly at Sarah's crib, staring at the sleeping newborn "with an almost hateful glare on his face."

Mr. and Mrs. Nelson took Marshall to see Dr. J. David, a psychologist specializing in children and families. An anxious Mrs. Nelson tells Dr. David of her concerns: "Between his sudden loss of bowel and bladder control, his trouble sleeping, and his tantrums, my husband and I are very concerned. . . . Frankly, I worry when I see the look on his face when he stands by Sarah's crib."

Mr. Nelson, looking anxious and out of place in this psychotherapist's office, adds, "Marshall was a happy child before Sarah came home. Maybe we should have prepared him better for her arrival?"

In the ensuing conversation, Dr. David learns that during Mrs. Nelson's pregnancy, neither parent spent much extra time with Marshall, and there was little discussion of the impending addition to the Nelson family. In fact, thinking that it might be upsetting to him, they avoided discussing how Sarah's birth would change things in the Nelson home.

Speaking to Marshall while the parents were in the waiting room, Dr. David confronted a squirming, uncomfortable, and oppositional three-year-old. "I hate her!" was Marshall's immediate response when asked how he liked his new sister. After fifteen minutes more, Dr. David had his assistant take Marshall to the play room while he met with the parents.

He explained that although they certainly didn't do anything wrong with Marshall during Mrs. Nelson's pregnancy, they also didn't involve Marshall in the impending birth of his sister. Marshall lacked a sense of participation in the event. He hadn't been prepared for the level of attention that would be needed by his sister, nor was he reassured that as her big brother, Marshall was a very important member of the family. After Sarah's birth, as the adult Nelsons' attention and time were naturally more focused on meeting her needs, the Nelsons had again not involved Marshall in Sarah's care.

Dr. David explained that as a result of all this, the natural level of jealousy that a three-year-old would feel on the arrival of a newborn sibling was increased many times. Though incorrect, Marshall saw the arrival of his sister as the beginning of the end of his relationship with his parents, especially with his mother. He felt as if he had been replaced in their affections.

In his eyes, Marshall saw the infant getting all his mother's attention; his father came home, said, "Hi, Marshall, how's it going, Son?" then picked up and played with a giggling Sarah, or, if she were asleep, sat and talked with Mother about all the wonderful things Sarah had done that day. Dr. David helped the Nelsons see how things looked to three-year-old Marshall—he felt abandoned, unloved, uncared for—and replaced by an infant!

Quickly understanding, a tearful Mrs. Nelson made the connection. "So Marshall started to act like an infant himself—wetting and soiling again—trying to get our attention back?" she asked. "And those temper tantrums were his way of saying, 'Hey, look at me,'" mused Mr. Nelson. Nodding, Dr. David added that Marshall's difficulty with sleep was another indication of his depression at being replaced.

In the following two months, Dr. David worked one-on-one with Marshall, using play therapy to help understand how Marshall actually felt and to enable Marshall to express his otherwise unacceptable feelings. Dr. David worked to teach Marshall how he could feel differently, actually nurturingly toward his sister. He had Mr. and Mrs. Nelson read several excellent books that discussed sibling rivalry and how to integrate a newborn into a family with children, then he discussed what they'd learned in several sessions with both parents. Marshall's parents and sister usually joined him near the end of each of his therapy sessions.

In this successful therapy, no medications were indicated or necessary. It required only several visits. Central to the therapy was Dr. David's understanding of the psychodynamics involved, as well as the Nelson's willingness to be educated about some other ways to deal more effectively with their son.

Behavioral Therapies

In contrast to psychodynamic therapy, behavioral therapies look at difficulties in life as being the result of bad habits. For example, various stimuli in the environment trigger specific responses that are maladaptive, rather than personal problems resulting from unconscious conflicts.

The goal of behavioral therapy is to unlearn and to revise certain actions, feelings, and thoughts. Behavioral therapists believe that the actions, feelings, and thoughts that need revising result from the individual having formed erroneous connections in his mind between certain occurrences and the meaning of those occurrences to that individual.

Perhaps the easiest way to understand behavioral therapy is to look at how it was developed and its basis. Conditioning—both *classical* and *operant*, as elucidated by the Russian physiologist Ivan Pavlov and the pioneering American experimental psychologists B. F. Skinner and John B. Watson—forms the early basis for work in behavioral therapy. Rather than look for meaning and the reasons for a specific action, behavioral therapists seek to examine what triggered that behavior.

Classical conditioning is a term familiar to most people educated in America; the now-famous work that Pavlov did with dogs is discussed in both college and high school psychology classes. Pavlov observed that hungry dogs started to salivate at the sight of meat they were about to be fed. By simultaneously ringing a bell as soon as the dogs saw the meat, he soon found that the dogs had come to associate the sound of the bell with the sight of the food. Most interestingly, he discovered that he was able to elicit salivation from the dogs solely by ringing the bell—they had been conditioned to associate the sound of the bell with the act of being fed.

In experiments performed by Skinner and Watson, it was learned that animals could be taught to perform certain behaviors on command or cue by causing a reinforcement to occur as a *consequence* of performing those behaviors. For example, a chimpanzee could be taught to press a certain button on a panel placed before him. By having the buttons set up so that a press on any of the "wrong" buttons had no effect and a press on the "right" button released a food pellet, the animal quickly learned to go from random strikes of the various buttons to intentionally pressing the right button to earn a food pellet. This is called *operant conditioning*.

An undesirable trait or behavior can be extinguished using these same techniques. Removing a favorite pastime or rewarding behavior that's different from the undesirable behavior can often motivate a child toward new and better behaviors. There are a number of techniques that are behavioral in origin. Many use relaxation as a base step, preparing the person to be more effective in the behavioral exercise to come.

Vicarious learning, or *modeling*, is often used to help a child overcome fear or to learn more effective behaviors in social settings. A child with a fear may watch another child do the feared activity or face the feared circumstance, then imitate the behavior as a way of quelling that fear in herself. A child with a problem in certain social situations may watch another child successfully deal with that problem, then imitate the behavior until he has mastered it for himself.

Desensitization is often used after relaxation periods, as is modeling. This technique is used to slowly introduce anxiety-producing situations to a child in a way that allows her to become comfortable and stay relaxed with circumstances that she previously could not tolerate. A child who was morbidly afraid of dogs, for example, could first talk about dogs. Then, pictures of various breeds of dogs might be shown to the child. Through a number of steps and over a period of time, the child would become desensitized to the fear of dogs. Of course, the size and nature of the steps and the period over which they are carried out would depend primarily on the individual child and her circumstances.

Flooding, self-management techniques, assertiveness training, behavioral rehearsal, and *social skills training* are all other behavioral therapies based on the same basic premise.

Token economies are often used in inpatient hospital settings, but they are also effective when used properly in the home. Token economies have proven helpful with many children in shaping and improving behavior. Indeed, behavioral therapies overall have proven to be extremely useful tools in modifying and improving behavior.

Cognitive Therapies

Cognitive therapies differ from psychodynamic therapy in that they focus primarily on symptoms rather than on unresolved, unconscious conflicts. They differ from behavioral therapies as well, concerned as they are with thoughts and the thought process instead of with behaviors.

Aaron Beck, a psychiatrist, originally developed cognitive therapy to treat patients with depression in the 1960s. Cognitive therapists believe that the way people think, their attitudes and basic assumptions about their world, determine how they feel about themselves, what they do, and how they act. Beck, and others who followed him, identified a number of errors in thinking—logical errors that appear valid on quick inspection but that cannot withstand careful scrutiny. Identifying these errors in thinking is a prime focus in cognitive therapy—helping the patients to see their distorted thinking and to identify how that thinking leads them to self-defeating behavior and difficult emotional states.

Cognitive therapy can work with children as well as adults. The only limiting factor is the emotional and intellectual maturity of the individual. Many of the abstractions inherent in identifying and explaining how logical errors in thought lead to difficult emotional states would be of little help to a preschool or school-aged child who is unable to appreciate them. Even so, adolescents and many precocious older children can benefit from this therapy.

Biological Therapies

Medical interventions, or *biological therapies*, are limited in this discussion to pharmacological treatments—the use of medications to help relieve symptoms of emotional and psychiatric problems.

If you determine that your child should be evaluated for therapy, it's likely that the person doing the evaluation will want the child to be seen by a physician for a medical evaluation as well. Many emotional or psychiatric illnesses can mimic physiological illnesses and vice versa. For example, the fatigue and apathy that can accompany a hypothyroid (low thyroid) condition can appear to be depression. Equally impressive, poor sleep, loss of appetite, random aches and pains, and irritability can all appear to be caused by a wide variety of physiological illnesses but may actually be signs of depression. The list of medical problems that can masquerade as psychiatric difficulties, and the list of psychiatric difficulties that can masquerade as medical problems are long and varied.

Often after a diagnosis is determined by any nonpsychiatric therapist, a consultation with a psychiatrist is recommended. This is to allow the psychiatrist to evaluate the child for possible treatment with medications, because many emotional and psychiatric difficulties respond well to medication.

Many difficulties experienced by children seem to be self-limiting, that is, they seem to "go away" as the children grow. Many others don't disappear with time but do respond well to the other therapies listed here and do not require medication.

Some of the emotional and psychiatric problems that children have, however, respond or respond far better only with the use of psychiatric medications. A good example of the range of treatment possibilities is seen by examining a large sample of children with a particular diagnosis. In a sample size of one thousand school-aged children with ADHD, a small number will be only mildly affected, the majority will be moderately affected, and another small number will be severely affected. The children only mildly affected may be able to achieve effectiveness in school and other situations by the use of behavioral modification techniques alone, perhaps combined with some cognitive work. The majority will benefit most from some behavioral (or behavioral and cognitive) therapy *and* stimulant medication. The severely affected will surely benefit from some behavioral and cognitive work, but the most important aspect of therapy for them will most likely be the stimulant medication. Several key points about medications should be kept in mind:

- Not all emotional or psychiatric problems require the use of medications

- Some problems will require medications only if present in moderate or severe forms

- Some problems will almost always require medications

- Psychotropic, or mood-altering, drugs should be prescribed only by a psychiatrist—either a general psychiatrist or one specializing in child and adolescent psychiatry

- Contrary to popular belief, psychiatric medication, properly prescribed and used, is almost never an addictive problem, even if the medication is one abused in the general population

- In modern psychiatric practice, children are *not* "drugged up"; for years, children and adults alike were often treated with medications that left them in a stupor; there simply were not many medications to choose from; today, however, if a medication leaves a child lethargic, the psychiatrist has many other medications (or combination of medications) to choose from that will control the symptoms but leave the child alert and functional

- Responsible psychiatrists *never* prescribe medications for the comfort or convenience of the parents or teachers; they use medication *only* when it will help the child in an important way

When discussing biological therapies, it is also important to acknowledge the roles genetic or medical problems play in bringing about your child's difficulties. Over the years—possibly in your childhood, certainly in that of your parents—many behaviors that were difficult, disruptive, and annoying were diagnosed as bad behaviors or even thought of as criminal. The children performing those behaviors were seen as committing those behaviors as if they were young criminals. Those children were called "bad," and their behaviors were "wrong" or even "evil"!

Yet discoveries in the last half of the twentieth century in the fields of brain chemistry, general psychiatry, neurology, psychopharmacology, and child and adolescent psychiatry have opened up new avenues of understanding, new ways of looking at old problems. There are several types of "good news" in these discoveries. The first is that you and your spouse may not have had anything to do with causing the problems that your child may experience.

For years in this country, an almost Victorian model held sway. If your child had problems, then you were a bad parent; at the least, you were ineffective. If you were a better parent, that model held, your child would be better behaved, more motivated, more normal. You, the parent, were to blame for your child's problems. If a child was "bad," it was because of poor parenting.

Even with the advances in understanding that have come, no one is going to suggest that parents needn't do the best job they can with their children. But for the first time, parents can realize that, although their job is important and they need to do the best they can, they don't need to be perfect parents to raise healthy, happy children! Indeed, even if they did everything right (which implies that all the experts could agree on what's right in every circumstance, which they clearly cannot), genetic predispositions and neurochemical problems that their children might have could cause difficulties nonetheless.

Moving people away from the moralistic view of behavior has proven difficult, but the situation is improving. For every teacher who believes that stricter discipline for the hyperactive child is the answer, many other teachers are just now realizing that ADHD is a *real* disorder, not a euphemism for a pain-in-the-neck kid. They're aware that the child can be treated and that yelling and humiliation don't work. If fact, it's quite the opposite. The more you yell, the more you humiliate, the angrier the child becomes—the anger is then acted out in unacceptable ways.

Just as everyone who has the gene for alcoholism does not become an alcoholic, not every child who has the genetic predisposition for one (or more) of the neurobiological disorders (NBDs) goes on to develop them. But some children do; and when they do, it's important that parents, teachers, and the children themselves (when they're ready) learn of these biologically determined difficulties.

Parents need to understand this so that they don't needlessly punish themselves with guilt for being poor parents when in fact they may have done a wonderful job. Teachers need to become educated about the NBDs; otherwise they risk making things worse for children who have one of these disorders by unfairly disciplining, punishing, or humiliating these children for behaviors and actions they cannot control without proper diagnosis and effective treatment.

As every parent knows or soon learns, children can be their own toughest critics. Care must be taken so that when children with these biologically determined problems are told of their disorder, they understand how treatment can make an important difference. Although many untreated disorders genuinely rob the child of the ability to behave differently, most disorders, with treatment, can no longer be used as excuses for inappropriate behavior.

In fact, just receiving the diagnosis may be therapeutic! What had been seen in the past as a moral failing, causing the child to suffer low self-esteem and a poor self-image, can now be seen as a medical problem. Of course, the child may still be held responsible for conscious choices he makes about his behavior. More important, though, is that the child no longer has to take responsibility for things that were always beyond his control. Instead, he can focus on how to achieve greater effectiveness in his life through appropriate treatment and education about the disorder.

Play Therapy and Family Therapy

Play therapy and *family therapy* are two important adjuncts to the other therapies we have discussed; either or both may be indicated in a child's situation.

Play therapy is most helpful in a circumstance in which the child being treated has difficulty expressing her emotions verbally because of her emotional and intellectual immaturity (as in the case of very young children), because the emotions developed are overwhelming or terrifying, or because the emotions are so embarrassing or humiliating that the child cannot bring herself to speak of them (for example, in the case of sexual abuse).

Engaging the child in play or observing the child at play lets the trained therapist, regardless of her professional designation, gain great insight into how the child processes information, how he relates to others, and the manner in which he regards himself. Using dolls and drawing implements, a therapist can elicit otherwise censored information—information, for instance, that the child might consciously censor for fear of retaliation by another child or an adult for "telling on them." Material that might otherwise be unconsciously censored (answers to questions at which the child "blanks out" perhaps because the repressed material is too horrible to deal with) may also be accessed.

Play therapy is not useful only for obtaining information, however. It can also convey important ideas. During play with the child, the therapist can demonstrate, with dolls or with imaginative stories, for example, philosophical concepts that might otherwise be too difficult for the child to grasp. Additionally, discussing some topics with a direct approach might be emotionally or intellectually too demanding for the child. Play therapy also allows the child to "test out" alternative ways of looking at her situation without confronting it directly, which might be too painful, too frightening, or just too overwhelming. Used by a well-trained, talented therapist, play therapy can be an extremely valuable tool for working with children.

Family therapy, much like its name implies, is therapeutic work done in the context of the whole family. Usually, of course, there is an *identified patient* here, a child. But, unlike one-on-one therapy in which there is just a patient and a therapist, here there is a therapist, an identified patient, and, if you will, copatients. The other members of the family are seen as part of the system in which the identified patient developed his symptoms. Hence, they are regarded as patients as well.

Family therapy relies on a *systems* approach to family dynamics, understanding the family as a dynamic whole that is comprised of discrete individuals, each being complete with his own feelings, personality, and history, yet also being part of a greater system, the family. The family also has its own feelings, personality, and history. Family therapists often refer to the family's culture, or ecology.

The (psycho)dynamic interplay of family members is examined by the therapist. In so doing, she gains a better understanding both of the individuals in that family and of the way that family operates. Otherwise unknown information, such as unspoken expectations, rules, rules enforcement, and manner and mode of relating between the family members becomes more apparent. This information can be helpful not just in helping heal the identified patient, but also in healing the copatients—and the family itself.

Family therapists use a variety of techniques for an assortment of problems and issues—techniques that are not a cure for the problems the family is experiencing but rather are the means to assist in facilitating the progress of the family. Some of these techniques, such as reframing, communication skill-building, family pictures, and genograms, are discussed next.

Reframing is taking a problem from one category and placing it into another category—changing it from being perceived as a negative to being perceived as a positive.

For instance, a teenager who is questioned about the use of the car every time she borrows it—where she went, what she did, and who rode in the car with her—may view such questions as a lack of trust on the parent's part. Reframing permits the questions to be viewed as a sign of caring and concern, if that is indeed what the parent is doing.

Communication skill-building. Communication deficits are apparent in many families, particularly in families in which one or more members may have attention deficit disorder, learning disorders, or other problems. These communication problems can prevent the family from functioning in a healthy manner.

A family therapist can teach family members how to listen to each other, how to restate issues or concerns, how to take turns stating opinions and feelings, how to argue fairly, and how to use the brainstorming techniques that allow members to toss out ideas freely, knowing they will not be judged personally for their thoughts.

The genogram. Another technique often used is the genogram. This is a schematic drawing representing the family tree on both sides of the child's family. Symbols are used to indicate male and female. The various members of both families, going back as many generations as possible (usually one or two) are labeled appropriately. The genogram is often sent with the parents as "homework" over several weeks. The tree is labeled with the emotional/psychiatric information available. Social data are also useful as clues to undiagnosed difficulties. Knowing that Uncle Joe drank a lot, had seventeen children by four wives, made and lost a million dollars—three times!—and died penniless might provide clues to make a therapist suspect that Uncle Joe might have had bipolar disorder.

Reducing thousands of words to a schematic drawing (the genogram) the therapist can quickly see the significant emotional history of the family and the relationship to the present difficulties being treated. The genogram also gives him a graphic tool to let his clients truly "see" what he's talking about, helping them to understand how they came to be the people they are. Understanding better how they became who they are can help them effect the change needed to become the people they'd like to be. Further, heritable traits that have caused difficulty can then be discussed with less guilt as the family sees the lines of transmission.

Family pictures reveal a wealth of information about family members, so their use in therapy is not surprising. Pictures uncover past and present dynamics of the family. When pictures are viewed together in a session with the family therapist, the responses and remarks that each family member makes or doesn't make, the excitement or lack of excitement when holiday or vacation pictures are viewed, and discussion of the reasons particular photographs were brought to the session permit the therapist to obtain a clearer picture of the family dynamics. This includes patterns of communication, and the role each member occupies in the family structure.

Used effectively, family therapy can range from helpful to crucial in dealing with the identified patient. It usually offers tremendous benefits to the other members of the family as well.

ELEVEN

The Continuum of Care

To reasonably determine what should be done for your child, it's important to know what *can* be done. In turn, understanding the philosophy and approach that motivate the people who practice the different therapies allows you to narrow the field even more.

Although the very nature of some kinds of therapy demands a specific setting, most can be implemented quite successfully in a wide range of settings. Understanding the *continuum of care* available—from weekly visits to a therapist's office to group therapy to full hospitalization—will help you get for your child the help he needs. Armed with knowledge of the levels of care available along this continuum, you and the therapist can look at your child's needs and determine what level of care will meet those needs most effectively.

Outpatient: Office or Clinic Setting

In this setting you, your child, or both of you will meet with the therapist, usually for fifty minutes to one hour. With very young children, this time will often be reduced to prevent fatigue. Outpatient therapy is the most frequently used therapeutic environment with a child, because its interference with the child's normal routine is minimal. The number of visits per week is usually adjustable to meet the child's needs. For a child having a difficult time with a special circumstance such as the serious illness of a parent or divorce, a therapist might call for multiple visits in the initial weeks.

In a stable therapeutic circumstance, one in which the child is doing well and is not suffering an acute impairment, she is often seen once a week or even once every two weeks as the work progresses. Of course, the therapist will see your child more often if you bring up a new concern or a worsening of an old one. It's not uncommon for a child who has been viewed as being greatly improved and doing well to occasionally slide back a step or two from time to time; it's part of the nature of personal growth.

In less stable circumstances, such as when a child is deemed to have a serious or life-threatening disturbance—one in which there is a risk of danger to self or others—the child will most likely be hospitalized. A depressed ten-year-old girl expressing suicidal thoughts or a teenage boy who has assaulted his teacher may need immediate hospitalization, for example. At the time of discharge, the physician, often a child and adolescent psychiatrist, will most likely want the child to continue the therapy that began in the hospital. The parents will probably be referred to a therapist who can see their child on an outpatient basis.

Beneficial both to some children who don't need hospitalization and to children immediately after hospitalization, outpatient therapy is also frequently used as the preferred setting for *supportive* therapy. The purpose of supportive therapy is to help those youngsters at great risk for recurrent hospitalization. In the case of chronically ill children with major psychiatric illnesses, delaying the need for hospitalization and shortening the ultimate hospital stay are worthwhile goals of this type of outpatient treatment. This is a form of outpatient treatment in which the patient is usually seen only once every month, or even every two months, during periods of relative remission. The frequency of visits, of course, is flexible and changes as the needs of the child change.

Case Management

A step further along the continuum of care, *case management* is used when a child needs extra help to live at home and in the community. In some communities the case manager has enormous resources available and can call on and coordinate the services of legal and financial consultants, as well as psychiatric and medical professionals to work with a child. In most communities, however, federal and state funding has been sharply reduced in recent years. As a result, many case managers carry a heavy case-load and do much of the work themselves. Still, a good case manager can be one of a child's most effective allies. If case management is suggested as an adjunct to treatment, it might prove helpful both to you and to your child.

Case management is often provided by a public health agency, usually at the county or parish level, but sometimes offered by state agencies. In response to the rising costs of revolving-door psychiatric admissions paid by private health insurers, case management is also offered by fee-for-service providers.

Keep in mind that case managers who work for public health agencies are often recent graduates working with that agency to gain experience. Even so, services provided are often top-notch. A private fee-for-service provider won't necessarily be able to do a better job. If case management is being offered to your child, ask your physician and therapist about the agency providing that service. They will often be able to tell you about the quality of the work.

Home-Based Treatment Program

This approach to treatment involves a team of specialists who go to the family home and work with both the child or adolescent and the rest of the family. The rationale here is that the person who evaluated the child felt that both the child and the whole family—parents and siblings alike—would benefit from some assistance. The child receives the immediate help he needs, while his parents learn more effective parenting skills. The child's siblings, too, are involved by the staff. This can serve a preventive and therapeutic purpose and often benefits everyone involved, leading to a better prognosis for families who are appropriate for this type of treatment program.

Day Treatment Program

Here the child has all the services available to him in a hospital, but the child goes home every day to rejoin his family. Special education services are part of this program, as are regular education programs. The child attends whichever is appropriate for him. Day treatment programs are usually set up for five-day-a-week attendance and are fairly intensive regimens. Children receive psychiatric care daily in a carefully controlled school environment.

Partial Hospitalization: Day Hospital

This is similar to a day treatment program in that all the services of a psychiatric hospital are available, but school services are not an integral part of the program. Like the day treatment program, this is an intensive therapeutic environment.

Emergency/Crisis Services

In communities that offer this service, twenty-four-hour-a-day psychiatric emergency services are available in a hospital emergency room. Many communities have extended these services by including mobile crisis teams who go to the patient for an on-site evaluation and intervention. Most often, these teams can also provide transport to the ER if that is deemed necessary. Many situations are appropriate for the use of a mobile crisis team. It's important, of course, to use discretion in calling a crisis center for assistance, but some circumstances always warrant their use. For example, anytime a child threatens to hurt themselves, to commit suicide, or to hurt anyone else, professional help should be sought immediately. If an emergency situation such as these arises when your usual mental health provider is not available, an immediate call to the crisis center is indicated. Be aware that many children, having said something "drastic" in the heat of argument and emotion, will recant as soon as they know the crisis center is being called. The temptation for most parents to relent and not to place the call can be strong. Unless you are absolutely satisfied with your own, very biased assessment of the situation, make the call. A child desperate enough to make the threat might just be desperate enough to follow through; get a professional assessment immediately.

A good rule of thumb to use in deciding whether to make the call or not is this: if something the child has done or said would result in physical harm to another if not interfered with, make the call. If something the child has done or said could cause serious emotional problems for another, especially another child, make the call. Lastly, if something the child has done or said frightens you for the well being of that child or anyone else, make the call.

Respite Care

Unlike the other programs listed here, respite care is for the benefit of the child or adolescent's primary caretaker, usually a parent. With the focus almost always on the child and his problems, the primary caretaker often gets short shrift. Because the caretaker is often shuffled to the side when the child is in crisis, many community mental health leaders have lobbied for respite care. They recognize that the role of a primary caretaker of a child with emotional or behavioral problems is an extremely taxing one. They also acknowledge the need for the caretaker to have a respite—to get a break. For even the most loving and concerned parent, several days, a week, or even just one day without the responsibility of caring for her child can be a godsend.

Not only do parents deserve that break, but also their childcare skills remain at a higher level if they are allowed an opportunity to rejuvenate and attend to their own needs. Here, specially trained staff take care of the child, out of the home, for periods ranging from one day to a week. This gives the primary caretaker the time to meet his own needs, relax, and revitalize.

Therapeutic Group Home or Group Residence

This type of program usually includes five to ten children or adolescents in a domicile staffed with personnel trained in attending to the psychiatric needs of children. Frequently these facilities are formally linked to a day treatment center or a specialized education facility. By their very nature they put emphasis on teaching socialization skills to children who often lack the ability to interact peacefully and effectively with others. These facilities are also useful for children who have had difficulty staying on a therapeutic regimen while in the home.

Crisis Residence

Here we find twenty-four-hour-a-day supervision in a locked facility. This is extremely valuable for the child who is acutely ill psychiatrically and who would otherwise risk becoming a danger to himself (suicidal) or to others. These residences usually provide crisis intervention and immediate acute treatment only, with an average stay from two or three days to ten days.

Residential Treatment Centers (RTCs)

Designed for seriously disturbed youth in need of long-term treatment, these facilities provide intensive, comprehensive, and ongoing psychiatric care. Most RTCs are established in a campus-like setting. To a casual passerby, the center would probably appear to be a boarding school. Indeed, educational facilities are an integral part of these centers.

Many such facilities are oriented to the care of a particular type of mental illness, with some specializing in the treatment of childhood schizophrenia, for example. Others specialize in the care of less pervasive illnesses. Still others provide care for a more general population of troubled children. Almost all of these facilities have accommodations and trained staff to deal with acutely difficult children or have arrangements with nearby psychiatric clinics or hospitals, should the need arise. Placements in RTCs are generally for longer-term care, with the shortest stay averaging a year or less.

Hospital Treatment

Hospitalization for more than a few days on a crisis-intervention basis may be indicated. At a psychiatric hospital, the child can receive the most intensive treatment and supervision available, usually with a greater choice of treatment modalities. The environment can be most carefully controlled in a hospital setting, which can be important in managing an acutely ill child.

As with several of the other types of care discussed, hospitalization can be expensive, often being the most expensive on a daily charge basis. With or without effective insurance coverage for this care, the family of the child will incur large expenses, so it's appropriate to discuss the child's needs with the admitting psychiatrist. What types of treatment will be provided and by whom? What is the anticipated length of stay and the total cost? What are the advantages of hospitalization here? What makes this the best choice for the treatment of my child? Are there alternatives that are less expensive but that would be just as effective for my child? If this was your child, where would you place her—and why?

In the end, the decision of where to place your child remains yours. By giving you a good idea of what is available in some communities, we hope we've given you help in making an intelligent, knowledgeable choice. Good choices are based on good information. Don't be afraid to ask questions.

In years gone by, many people were intimidated by medical personnel, especially by physicians. Don't be! You, your child, and your child's doctor are partners in your child's mental health care—full partners! Although it's true that your child might not be fully able to participate in the decision-making process, you are, and you must. If a therapist or physician wants to use a therapy, a medication, or a placement for your child that you don't understand, insist that you be given an accurate explanation that you can comprehend.

No ethical therapist or physician should object to your obtaining a second opinion; if you are uneasy about the recommendations of your child's therapist or physician, we urge you to obtain one.

Unfortunately, your love and concern for your child often are not enough to help him when he's truly ill. Fortunately, your love and concern, and the knowledge you possess about your child, are important assets to him—assets that can guide you in your choice of professionals, therapies, and treatment settings.

TWELVE

Their Future, Your Past

If you are a caring and concerned parent, you want the best that life has to offer your child. You want to provide a stable and consistent home environment and be able to provide the best education for your child. You want what most parents want for their children: happiness, love, and success.

When a child has an emotional or behavioral problem, most parents want to help in any way they can. They hurry over to school to see what the problem is; they make an appointment to talk to their child's physician or take the child to a psychiatrist; or they read a book to learn ways to relate to their child. But what many parents fail to do is to take a good look at themselves and the home environment. Yes, sometimes a child's problems are made worse, or even begin, right at home. Then they are carried out the front door into the world. We are *not* saying you are to blame for your child's problems—unless you are guilty of neglect and abuse. What we are saying is this: Your well-intended parenting style may actually exacerbate some of your child's problems. No parent is perfect, and even good parents can become better parents. If you think your child needs therapy, or if your child is in therapy, changes in the family environment will only help, not hinder, your child's improvement.

How Home Life Can Interfere with a Child's Life

There's been a lot of talk lately in the media about famous people who have grown up in dysfunctional families. So much talk, in fact, that now the general public is asking, "Who *hasn't* grown up in a dysfunctional family?"

We all bring positive attributes from childhood into adulthood, but we also bring with us some negative attributes (excess baggage, we like to call them). It's the excess baggage that we address in this chapter because it often can prevent us from being the best parents we are capable of being. Hopefully, this chapter will open your eyes to some thoughts that you might not have considered before. So later in the chapter we'll throw out some questions for you to contemplate further.

How One Family Came to Be

We are unique individuals with our own personalities and temperaments—that's why one person who is angry and upset can count to ten before calmly replying, while another person immediately explodes. A person who explodes can be taught to respond in a different manner, like counting to ten first. The calm person, if continuously pushed, can learn to explode. But just as we were born with our own temperaments, we were also born into a specific family. If we were raised in a family of five, we then had four other distinct personalities and temperaments to live with—all of which had some effect on us.

How we were raised, how family members reacted and related to each other, whether we had a sibling with a disability, a parent who drank too much, a consistently unemployed father, an abusive mother, a domineering parent, or good, loving parents—all of these factors made an impact on us, forming us into the unique individuals we are today.

To demonstrate how all of this works, we'll present to you the Smith family, a family of three.

Sherry the Child

Sherry's mother was a perfectionist, just like her own mother, Sherry's grandmother—everything had a place in the home, and there was no excuse for anything being out of place. The upstairs was cleaned on Thursday, the downstairs on Friday. The wash was done on Monday, the ironing on Tuesday. Sherry was never embarrassed to bring a friend into her home; it was always immaculate. But few friends wanted to be in the atmosphere of Sherry's home.

Sherry's dad traveled frequently. Although her father was a kind and loving man, he felt he had little to say about the way Sherry's mother ran the home.

Sherry's mother never talked with Sherry about anything; she never asked Sherry about school or her friends, her thoughts, feelings, or ideas. Not only was Sherry's perfectionist mother unavailable emotionally to her, but she was also very strict. Mom made all the decisions and all the rules. Sherry never had to make a decision about anything. As a result, Sherry grew up with low self-esteem; she worried about things that she thought she had no control over; she couldn't ever make a decision without a great deal of thought so she didn't make decisions. She would allow others to make decisions for her. She became withdrawn and depressed. Not understanding all of the dynamics involved in her childhood, especially her relationship with her mother and the effect this would ultimately have on her, Sherry was very vulnerable to meet a man like Ken Smith.

Ken the Child
Ken's mother also was domineering—she ran the family and controlled the finances—much like Sherry's mom. But Ken handled it differently. Rather than abide by the rules as Sherry did, Ken rebelled and made his own rules. His attitude got him into a lot of trouble in his mid- and late-teen years, and eventually he was thrown out of the private school he attended. His parents always bailed him out of trouble. A somewhat overweight and arrogant teenager, Ken ran with the wrong crowd because it was the only crowd who accepted him. Not surprisingly, his self-esteem was poor. By age seventeen, he was working part-time to support a gambling habit. He learned to lie, manipulate, and use people. At age twenty-five, he stopped gambling and decided to get his act together.

With one failed marriage behind him, at age thirty-two, Ken, fell into a marvelous career opportunity and became quite wealthy and successful. His life had changed, but Ken had not. He was still Ken, the rebel, the master of manipulation, the controller. He still lived by his own rules, cheating and lying to people whenever he had the opportunity. Ken also liked money and the power it brought him—so much, in fact, that he thought money could buy anything and anybody. Money was both power and control, Ken believed; it could buy love, even happiness. Not surprisingly, Ken was attracted to Sherry.

Sherry and Ken (Husband and Wife, Mother and Father)

Sherry and Ken married. Sherry needed someone to take care of her, to tell her what to do, and how to do it. Ken, on the other hand, needed someone to control and he controlled Sherry. Sherry thought this was normal because her mother had also controlled her. Ken was generous, and he showed his love by providing Sherry with the best of everything. Sherry did as Ken asked, never considering her own needs. Before long, the couple had a child together.

Sherry had a wonderful relationship with her son. She did believe that children need to be disciplined, but unlike her mother, who was very strict and overly protective, she disciplined fairly. A messy home disturbed her (not surprisingly), and Ken and she would argue about the house occasionally. She also called Ken on his lies on occasion, but not consistently because she was afraid of Ken, just as she had always been of her mother.

Because of Ken's indifference to rules, he was more apt to let his son get away with things. Often knowingly, he would sabotage some of Sherry's attempts at discipline. Whereas Sherry showed her love to the child by spending time with him, Ken bought his love with the latest gadgets and toys.

Their son, Kevin, who is thirteen, is much like Ken. He exhibits emotional and behavioral problems at home and in school, plus he has little respect for authority figures. Yet, talking with Kevin, ones finds that his mother's influence was not entirely wasted. The problem for Kevin is that he's been struggling between two different value systems. Mom stresses to tell the truth and to follow the rules. Dad is a hard worker, but he often lies and shows by his own actions that rules are meant to be broken. Kevin is learning from his father that money, power, and control are important.

Both Ken and Sherry brought some good qualities into the marriage, but they also brought a tremendous amount of baggage from their childhood, including their own insecurities and low self-esteem. And that's the point of this story. We often have baggage that interferes with our relationships, but most importantly, without our knowledge that baggage can interfere with the way we raise our children.

Kevin

Until a child begins to break his dependence from them, his most important role models are his parents. He learns by example what is right and wrong, how to resolve conflicts, and how to express anger, happiness, sadness, joy, kindness, and so forth. If, for instance, his parents are concerned about people in their community who are in need of food and he participates in taking food to people's homes, he learns the importance of helping people in need. However, if he watches a parent steal small items from a store, he learns that stealing is okay as long as you don't get caught. When a man beats his wife, or the wife makes demeaning remarks to her husband, the child learns that it's okay to be abusive.

Put yourself in Kevin's place. From one parent he hears that lying is wrong and that true happiness is not monetary. From the other parent he learns that lying and using people are not only okay, but also the road to success. To Kevin, his dad seems more forceful, more successful than his mother.

At times, Kevin feels guilty—he loves his mother and his father, but he feels torn. Inside he knows that his dad's actions are not right, "but just look at my dad! He's so successful that he can buy anything he wants, do anything he wants. I mean, he's got power!" Dad's influence has been much stronger than Mom's so far. Kevin is also an angry boy who is confused and depressed, and he has begun acting out his frustrations both in the home and at school.

But There's More to the Story

Kevin has attention deficit hyperactivity disorder and learning disorders. Because of his disabilities and his own temperament (aggressive, outspoken, a loner, somewhat depressed, with little regard for authority), he also shows symptoms of oppositional defiant disorder and is at risk for developing conduct disorder. Even worse, he is at great risk for becoming antisocial, just like his father.

We can't predict how Kevin will turn out, but we have our thoughts. Without professional intervention, without Kevin's parents working toward the same goals—providing a united front and being seen as equals—Kevin is going to have a tough time in life. Before we can expect to see any changes in Kevin, his parents must make some changes in the home and in their attitudes; otherwise Kevin will continue his acting-out behaviors. Placing a child like Kevin into weekly therapy sessions, no matter how well intended, will not produce the positive results one should expect as long as Kevin returns to the same home environment day after day.

We are by no means suggesting that Kevin be removed from the home. We are stressing the importance of family dynamics and the tremendous long-term effect they can have on a growing child. For this family to help Kevin, both Mom and Dad need therapy also.

What about That Baggage?

We all have baggage from our past that influences our actions and our relationships. That does not mean that we are bad people or that we are bad parents. Nor does it mean we are the cause of our child's difficulties. That baggage didn't just happen to us. We didn't acquire it on our own. Remember that it is a combination of our own temperaments, the way we were raised, how our parents reacted, how we reacted, environment, and genetics— and it is also a series of other life events and relationships that we have experienced over the years that makes us the people we are today.

We have the power within ourselves to face the baggage and to make changes that will benefit our children. Change is always difficult, though, and never as easy as it sounds. It takes parents with a commitment to the same goal, parents willing to look at their own behaviors and to admit that change is needed. In some cases, change can occur only when parents are willing to expose and trust themselves and their family to the intervention of a mental health professional—because only then can the family become healthy and whole.

In any family in which even one member is having difficulties, the entire family is affected. A parent who has a drinking problem or suffers from depression has an effect on the entire family. A child with an emotional, behavioral, or learning disorder also affects the entire family.

Take a look at yourself. Can you identify any situations from your past that may have resulted in excess baggage?

Here are a few questions that might jog some memories. Check off those questions that remind you of yourself in your relationship with your child or a situation in your home today. Those areas *may* be causing conflict in your home and adversely affecting your child without anyone in the home even being aware of the damage to the child.

Your Parents during Your Childhood

- Was there physical, sexual, or emotional abuse during your childhood? Were either of your parents abused in his or her childhood?

- Did one of your parents suffer from depression or any other psychiatric illness?

- Were your parents overly protective? Too strict? Or did you pretty much do what you wanted because there were no rules?

- Did you have a parent who was domineering, a perfectionist, or never around?

- Were you constantly compared to a sibling?

- Did your parents have financial problems that caused a great deal of stress?

- Did your parents argue a lot?

- Did your parents divorce when you were a child?

- Did one of your parents spend a great deal of time in the hospital?

- Did you spend a lot of time with baby-sitters or other caretakers?

- Did one parent make all the decisions, enforce the rules, handle all of the discipline?

- Did your parents make time for you? Or was something else always more important?

- Did they talk with you? Listen when you came to them with problems or questions? Share in your happiness? Ask about your day?

- Do you feel that your parents expected too much from you? Or maybe even too little?

- Did you feel like your best was never quite good enough? Did anyone ever tell you that you could do better if you only tried harder? Could you have done better? If so, what got in your way?

- Did either of your parents have a substance abuse problem?

- Did either parent commit suicide?

- Did one of your parents die when you were a child?

Siblings

- Were you afraid of one of your siblings?

- Did one sibling demand more of your parents' time than you received from them?

- Did you have a chronically ill sibling?

- Did you lose a sibling to death during your childhood?

- Did one of your siblings have a physical, emotional, or behavioral problem?

Home and School

- Did your parents help you with schoolwork?

- Did your parents come to school activities such as parent-teacher conferences, plays, or sports that you were involved in?

- Were you permitted to have friends visit your home?

- Did your friends enjoy coming to your home?

- Were you ever included in making family decisions regarding house rules, curfews, household purchases, family outings, or vacations?

- Did you feel like an important and contributing member of your family?

- Did your parents believe children should be seen but not heard?

- Did your parents sit and talk *with* you, not "at" you? Did you feel like you could go to your parents with any problems and they would drop what they were doing to sit and listen?

- When you finally left home (either to marry or live on your own), did you feel confident, responsible, able to make your own decisions?

- At what age do you think you finally reached adulthood? (Some people leave home feeling like an adult, others never feel like an adult until their mid-thirties, forties, or even later.)

Now Let's Take a Look at Today

- Do you have a happy feeling inside when you think about your childhood? Or do you feel sad, cheated, disappointed, abandoned, or indifferent? Do you remember much about your childhood? If not, why do you think that is the case?

- Do you have any problems with abusing drugs?

- Do you have any psychological, psychiatric, or learning problems (depression, antisocial behaviors, attention deficit disorder, learning disorder, panic attacks, anxiety disorder, et cetera)?

- Are you domineering, a perfectionist, abusive?

- Are you happy being married? Happy being a single parent?

- Do you have outside activities that delight you?

- Do you have an ailing parent who needs your help frequently, if not always?

- Do you have time during the day just for you?

- Do you feel like your children demand more than you can give?

- Do you ever wish you could just run off and never return to your family?

- Does your spouse agree with you on how to discipline the children?

Looking at the Past Can Help with Today

Usually the problems we grew up with in childhood are carried into adulthood unless we recognized the problems early and received professional intervention to assist us with overcoming obstacles from our past. For instance, do you ever find yourself saying something to your son or daughter, and then cringing inside and thinking, "My mother (or father) used to say that, and I swore I never would." Are you actively trying to change the remarks that "just come out" of your mouth? Unkind words or hurtful statements, sometimes said in jest but said just the same, can cause emotional damage to children. Remember the saying, "Sticks and stones may break my bones, but words will never harm me"? What fool wrote those words? Broken bones heal; words are remembered forever. A child who is told he is stupid or lazy will believe he is stupid or lazy. And a child who is told she is kind, goodhearted, and a great friend to others will believe just that.

If your parents spent little time with you as you were growing up, are you doing the same with your children? When is the last time you took an entire day—sunrise to sunset—and spent that time sharing activities with your children? (We're not talking about vacations here, but rather about taking a day now and then and giving it to your children doing something they would like.) Do you set aside some time every day to sit down and talk with your children individually? It doesn't have to be a long time—even fifteen to thirty minutes a day, or every other day, can strengthen your relationship with your children immensely and increase their self-esteem.

Do you believe that your marriage may be causing problems for your children? If so, what can *you* change so that it is not as stressful for your children? Can you spend more time with them? Do you address their feelings about what is going on in the home? Have you considered seeking help from a mental health professional as a family?

Sometimes our ideas of discipline are different from those of our spouse. Sometimes our values are different from each other's. Sometimes what we believe to be needed, like a clean house and nice dinners, is not what our children need. Are you putting too much emphasis on unimportant issues? Have you and your spouse talked about your differences in disciplining the children? Have you tried to reach a consensus? If you are not in agreement, you can unknowingly sabotage the efforts of each other. Children need routines, structure, and consistent discipline. They need to know what is expected of them to feel secure. Inconsistent discipline can be detrimental to any child. Without a united parental front, children are apt to play one parent against the other or to assume that the rules are not really important because even Mom and Dad can't agree on them.

We all hear our children talking, but do you really listen to what they are saying? Or are you too busy? Instead of hearing the opening phrases of your child's problems, forming an opinion of what the trouble is, and providing a quick solution, just sit quietly and really listen to your child. Be there for your child, so that with careful listening and skilled observation, you can truly understand what's important to her and what she is actually telling you.

Have you ever thought that maybe your style of disciplining is in direct conflict with the temperament of your child? How does he react to threats? Some children, at the mere thought of losing something, instantly comply. Others don't. How does she react to a raised voice? Again, some children immediately mind; others do not. The thought of punishment is enough for some children, whereas other children need to work toward rewards and privileges. Children who cannot handle transitions easily must be warned that a change is about to occur. Other children do not need to be warned. It's imperative that you work with your child to find what motivates him. It takes a conscientious parent to find which techniques work best with a specific child.

Other Ways You Can Change Your Approach

Are there other ways you can change to help you deal with your child more effectively? Here are some possibilities, but the list is not limited just to those noted here. Use your imagination.

- Consider changing your reactions to behaviors that you are having difficulty dealing with; children quickly learn how we will respond to a particular situation, what buttons to push, and they sometimes say or do something inappropriate just to get our reaction; try defusing the situation with humor the next time; or try whispering your response

- Be more understanding; as we mentioned, listen and hear what your child is saying and don't jump to conclusions; if your child says he's sad, don't ask why; instead try this: "I hear you telling me that you are sad. What can I do to help? Can you tell me about it?"; identify with his feelings because they are real

• Watch his body language; he may be saying one thing to you, but his body language may be saying something else; question gently

• Show an interest in him and what is important to him; asking, "How was the game today?" while you are in the next room cleaning the toilet doesn't count

• A child who is experiencing any type of difficulty needs to know he is loved and valued; when was the last time you assured your son that he is loved, cherished, appreciated, and important to you?

• Permit him to have friends over for dinner, just to play for the day or to spend the night; children like to share their family and home with their friends and to show off their prized possessions; this also gives you the opportunity to observe their social skills

• Provide lots of encouragement and support; emphasize strengths (talents and interests) instead of weaknesses; children with emotional or behavioral difficulties need to know you are in their corner

• Negotiate rules; your children are more apt to cooperate if they have had an opportunity to help make the rules and help decide the consequences of breaking the rules

• Keep your expectations realistic; a child with learning disorders or ADHD, severe behavioral problems, and so forth, may never do as well in school as her peers, even though she may be just as bright; learn to accept your child and her difficulties; strive for improvement, not perfection

• Respect your child; she will not respect you unless the respect is returned

Parenting the Child with Behavioral or Emotional Problems

Parenting children with challenges is a demanding job for any parent, no matter how competent. Recognizing the areas that our children are struggling in and finding ways to help—while acknowledging, encouraging, and supporting them to recognize and appreciate their strengths, talents, and interests—are important aspects of parenting. It takes a firm commitment, a united parental front, changes in our approach to parenting, sometimes a change in schools or grade placement, adherence to medication schedules and therapy, but most of all it takes the ability to accept the child—challenges and all.

Accepting the Child

It is ironic that parents often demand that their children conform to certain standards—often the same standards that even we as adults cannot meet. We oftentimes try to exert power and control, to dominate their very thoughts and actions—especially if they are in direct conflict with what we believe to be correct or socially acceptable.

We must accept that children are children, with their own thoughts, likes, dislikes, feelings, attitudes, preferences, eccentricities, strengths, and weaknesses. Would we dare tell our best friend how to think or feel? Yet we do this with our children. "Don't cry," we say to our little boy. It doesn't matter that he cries from the pain of words, or that he hurts from the loss of a friendship or from a skinned knee, or that he cries because he feels different from other boys his age. What matters is that he hurts, and the concerned parent reaches out wanting to know about that hurt—helping him express that hurt verbally. It is usually difficult for children to express their feelings because they often lack the knowledge and vocabulary or because they keep their feelings locked up inside.

So, what else do we mean by accepting your child? The child with Tourette's disorder, obsessive-compulsive disorder, or attention deficit disorder, for instance, may display behaviors that are not considered "socially acceptable." Medications, therapy, parental guidance, and behavior modification can be extremely helpful. We can modify behaviors, but some things, such as the child's temperament or the fact that she has a disability, we cannot change. We can expect only what our child is capable of delivering. And sometimes that interferes with our expectations and those of society. We must adjust our expectations to meet our child's strengths and weaknesses, paying particular attention to his strengths. If we don't, we haven't accepted our child, and his struggles will be far worse than they need to be.

Learning to Cope

The effects of any emotional, behavioral, or learning disorder ripple outward from the child to family, friends, and peers at home and school. The child is often referred to as stupid, crazy, lazy, or worse. Often the child sees himself as "different" or "stupid." Most children with a disorder know they are different. Although they often cannot explain why, they know how they feel inside, and it's often a feeling of shame. That shame may cause them to act out in various ways, ranging from withdrawal to physical aggression. Their disorder may produce social awkwardness or social skills deficits, so they may have trouble making or keeping friends. They may also struggle in school, at sports, or within the family environment.

Without professional intervention, the situation can spiral out of control. The more frustrated children become, the more they fail—and the more they act out. The more they act out, the more they provoke and the more punishment they must endure—further damaging their already lowered self-esteem.

A child with a disorder can be an emotional burden to the family. Siblings can become jealous of the attention the child receives, or they might be annoyed or embarrassed by their sibling. Parents may feel like they are on an emotional treadmill as they struggle through a spectrum of emotions: frustration, denial, indignation, blame, guilt, and despair.

Therapy can help both the child and other family members, giving them the opportunity to vent their feelings while receiving support and reassurance. For the affected child, a more positive attitude about her own capabilities can be attained as she acquires insight into her own strengths and learns to cope with her disorder.

As parents, you travel a frightening road with a child who is suffering from a disorder, but you are never alone. No matter the type of challenge your child is facing, no matter how helpless you may feel, know that other parents like you are traveling the same road. It is from these families that you can draw strength and comfort, unearth effective ways to cope, obtain advice, and learn new parenting strategies that will make your job as parents a little easier, a little lighter.

Mental health professionals can help your child. Community and national organizations and local parent support groups can provide additional information and assistance. The information and the assistance are there to help you help your child. You need only to reach out to others.

Afterword

The mental health of your child is extremely important; it affects the way the child perceives herself and others around her. Just as important to note is that a child's mental health is important at every stage of her development, helping her to form opinions, make decisions, and handle the everyday stress she encounters. A child may be mentally healthy at one stage of development but not so healthy at another stage due to any number of circumstances, including school, personal and family relationships, and the child's physical health.

When a child's mental health is compromised, it interferes with the way the child thinks, feels, and acts. In other words, it interrupts the child's developmental stage. When a problem is not recognized, diagnosed, and treated, the fallout can lead to such things as drug abuse, academic failure, problems with personal relationships, family conflict, aggressive behaviors (acting out), criminal activities, and even suicide. The repercussions may also compromise the child's adult years—indeed, the effects can last a lifetime!

Although most parents cannot diagnose a specific mental health problem, they are capable of recognizing the signs that indicate that the child requires help. And that is what we hope this book has provided for you—the ability to recognize the signs that may suggest a child is experiencing an emotional, behavioral, or learning problem. This ability to identify possible mental health problems when they appear may help to keep them from becoming much worse in the future. Prompt intervention is extremely important.

If your child is struggling, it behooves you to seek help immediately. Search for as much information as you can about the mental health services that are available in your community, including case management, family support, parent training programs, outreach teams, day treatment, highly concentrated family-based counseling, residential care, foster care, respite care for parents, local support groups for a particular disorder formed by other parents, special education services, tutoring, vocational counseling for teenagers, and legal services. Information can be found from hotlines, libraries, the Internet, professionals, other parents in your community, and the national organizations listed in this book. Knowledge is empowering. It gives you support, strength, and competence. It can make the difference between a child being effectively treated and a child receiving mediocre treatment.

Appendices

NATIONAL ORGANIZATIONS

Alliance for the Mentally Ill
432 Park Ave., S., #710
New York, NY 10016
(212) 684-3264 (helpline)

Alliance of Genetic Support Groups
35 Wisconsin Circle, Suite 440
Chevy Chase, MD 20815
(800) 336-4363 (voice)

American Academy of Child and Adolescent Psychiatry
3615 Wisconsin Ave., NW
Washington, DC 20016
(202) 966-7300 (voice)
(800) 333-7636 (voice)

American Academy of Pediatrics
141 Northwest Pt. Blvd.
PO Box 927
Elk Grove Village, IL 60009
(708) 228-5005 (voice)
(708) 228-5097 (fax)

American Anorexia/Bulimia Association
c/o Regent Hospital
425 E. 61 St.
New York, NY 10021
(212) 891-8686 (voice)

American Association for Marriage and Family Therapy
1133 15th St., NW, Suite 300
Washington, DC 20005
(202) 452-0109 (voice)

American Association of Psychiatric Services for Children
1200C Scottsville Rd., Suite 225
Rochester, NY 14624
(716) 235-6910 (voice)

American Association of Suicidology
4201 Connecticut Ave., NW, Suite 310
Washington, DC 20008
(202) 237-2280 (voice)
(202) 237-2282 (fax)

American Hospital Association
840 Lake Shore Dr.
Chicago, IL 60611
(312) 280-6000 (voice)

American Occupational Therapy Association
1383 Piccard Dr.
PO Box 1725
Rockville, MD 20850-0822

American Psychiatric Association
1400 K St., NW
Washington, DC 20005
(202) 682-6000 (voice)

American Psychological Association
750 First St., NE
Washington, DC 20005
(202) 336-5500 (voice)

American Sleep Disorders Association
1610 14th St., NW, Suite 300
Rochester, MN 55901
(507) 287-6006 (voice)

American Speech-Language-Hearing Association
10801 Rockville Pike
Rockville, MD 20852
(800) 638-8255 (consumer helpline)
(301) 897-5700 (voice/TTY)
(301) 571-0457 (fax)

Anxiety Disorders Association of America
6000 Executive Blvd., Suite 513
Rockville, MD 20850
(301) 231-9350 (voice)

Association for the Care of Children's Health
7910 Woodman Ave., Suite 300
Bethesda, MD 20814
(301) 654-6549 (voice)
(800) 808-2224 (voice)

Association of American Medical Colleges
2450 N St., NW
Washington, DC 20037
(202) 828-0400 (voice)
(202) 828-1125 (fax)

Autism Network International
PO Box 448
Syracuse, NY 13201

Autism Services Center
PO Box 507
Huntington, WV 25710-0507
(304) 525-8014 (voice)

Autism Society of America
7910 Woodmont Ave., Suite 655
Bethesda, MD 20814
(301) 657-0881 (voice)
(800) 328-8476 (voice)

Canadian Mental Health Association
2160 Yonge St., 3rd Floor
Toronto, Ontario, Canada M4S 2Z3

Canadian Psychiatric Association
237 Argyle Ave., Suite 200
Ottawa, Ontario, Canada K2P 1B8

Center for Mental Health Services Knowledge Exchange Network (KEN)
PO Box 42490
Washington, DC 20015
(800) 789-2647
(301) 984-8796 (fax)
(301) 443-9006 (TDD)

Center for the Study of Anorexia and Bulimia
1 West 91st St.
New York, NY 10024
(212) 595-3449 (voice)

Child Welfare League of America, Inc.
440 1st St., NW
Washington, DC 20001
(202) 638-2952 (voice)

Children with Attention Deficit Disorders (CHADD)
499 N.W. 70th Ave., Suite 308
Plantation, FL 33317
(305) 587-3700 (voice)

Council for Exceptional Children
11920 Association Dr.
Reston, VA 22091
(703) 620-3660 (voice)
(703) 264-9446 (TTY)
(703) 264-9474 (fax)

Eating Disorders Awareness and
Prevention, Inc.
603 Stewart St., Suite 803
Seattle, WA 98101
(206) 382-3587 (voice)
(206) 292-9890 (fax)

Education Resources Information
Center (ERIC)
1920 Association Dr.
Reston, VA 22091
(703) 620-3660 (voice)

ERIC Clearinghouse on
Handicapped and Gifted Children
Council for Exceptional Children (CEC)
1920 Association Dr.
Reston, VA 22091-1589
(800) 438-8841 (voice)

Family Resource Center on
Disabilities
200 East Jackson Blvd., Room 900
Chicago, IL 60604
(312) 939-3513 (voice)
(312) 939-3519 (TDD)
(800) 952-4199 (voice)

Federation for Children with
Special Needs
95 Berkeley St., Suite 104
Boston, MA 02116
(617) 482-2915 (voice)
(617) 695-2939 (fax)

Foundation for Children with
Learning Disabilities
99 Park Ave.
New York, NY 10016
(212) 687-7211 (voice)

Health Care Financing
Administration
200 Independence Ave., SW
Room 428-H
Washington, DC 20201
(202) 690-7159 (fax)
(202) 690-6978 (voice)

Information Center for
Individuals with Disabilities
Information Specialist
Ft. Point Place
27-43 Wormwood St.
Boston, MA 02210-1606
(617) 727-5540 (voice)
(800) 462-5015 (voice in Maryland)
(617) 345-5318/9743 (fax/TDD)

Learning Disabilities Association
of America
4156 Library Rd.
Pittsburgh, PA 15234
(412) 341-1515 (voice)

Mental Illness Foundation
420 Lexington Ave., Suite 2104
New York, NY 10170
(212) 682-4699 (voice)

National Academy for
Child Development
PO Box 380
Huntsville, UT 84317
(801) 621-8606 (voice)
(801) 621-8389 (fax)

National Alliance for
the Mentally Ill
200 N. Glebe Rd., Suite 1015
Arlington, VA 22201
(800) 950-NAMI (helpline)
(703) 524-7600 (voice)
(703) 516-7991 (TDD)
(703) 524-9094 (fax)

National Alliance for Research on
Schizophrenia and Depression
60 Cutter Mill Rd., Suite 200
Great Neck, NY 11021
(516) 829-0091 (voice)
(516) 487-6930 (fax)

National Association for
Down Syndrome
PO Box 4542
Oak Park, IL 60522
(708) 325-9112 (voice)

National Association for
Self-Esteem
1775 Sherman St., Suite 1515
Denver, CO 80203
(800) 488-NASE (voice)

National Association of Anorexia
Nervosa and Associated Disorders
1936 Green Bay Rd.
Highland Park, IL 60035
(708) 432-8000 (voice)

National Association of Private
Schools for Exceptional Children
1522 K St., NW, Suite 1032
Washington, DC 20005
(202) 408-3338 (voice)

National Association of
Social Workers
750 First St., NE, Suite 700
Washington, DC 20002
(202) 408-8600 (voice)
(202) 836-8310 (fax)
(800) 638-8799 (voice)

National Association of
Therapeutic Wilderness Camps
4270 Hambrick Way
Stone Mountain, GA 30083
(404) 508-1036 (voice)
(404) 508-1514 (fax)

National Clearinghouse on
Alcohol and Drug Information
PO Box 2345
Rockville, MD 20847
(800) 729-6686 (voice)

National Committee for
Citizens in Education
410 Wide Lake Village Green
Columbia, MD 21044
(800) NETWORK (voice)

National Council on Stuttering
2136 West Agatite St.
Chicago, IL 60625
(312) 878-9717 (voice)

National Crisis Prevention
Institute
3315K N. 124th St.
Brookfield, WI 53005
(414) 783-5787 (voice)
(800) 558-8976 (voice)

National Depressive and Manic
Depressive Association
730 N. Franklin St., Suite 501
Chicago, IL 60610-3526
(800) 82-NDMDA (voice)
(312) 642-0049 (voice)
(312) 642-7243 (fax)

National Down Syndrome
Congress
1605 Chantilly Dr., Suite 250
Atlanta, GA 30324
(404) 633-1555 (voice)
(800) 232-NDSC (voice)

National Foundation for
Depressive Illness
PO Box 2257
New York, NY 10116
(212) 268-4260 (voice)
(800) 248-4344 (voice)

National Information Center for
Children and Youth with
Disabilities (NICHY)
PO Box 1492
Washington, DC 20013
(800) 695-0285 (voice)
(202) 884-8200 (voice)

National Institute of Child Health
and Human Development
Building 31, Room 2A32
9000 Rockville Pike
Bethesda, MD 20892
(310) 496-5133 (voice)

National Institute of Mental
Health (NIMH), Panic Disorder
Education Program
5600 Fishers Lane, Room 7C-02
Rockville, MD 20857
(301) 443-4513 (voice)
(800) 64- PANIC (voice)
(301) 443-8431 (TDD)

National Institute on Deafness and
Other Communicative Disorders
1 Communication Ave.
Bethesda, MD 20892-3456
(800) 241-1044 (voice)
(800) 241-1055 (TDD/TT)
(800) 907-8830 (fax)

National Mental Health
Association
1021 Prince St.
Alexandria, VA 22314-2971
(703) 684-7722 (voice)
(800) 969-6642 (voice)
(703) 684-5968 (fax)

New Jersey Center for Outreach
and Services for the Autism
Community, Inc.
1450 Parkside Ave., Suite 22
Ewing, NJ 08638
(609) 883-8100 (voice)
(800) 428-8476 (helpline New Jersey
only)
(609) 883-5509 (fax)

Obsessive Compulsive Foundation,
Inc.
PO Box 70
Milford, CT 06460
(203) 878-5669 (voice)
(203) 874-2826 (fax)
(203) 874-3843 (infoline)

Orton Dyslexia Society
Chester Building, Suite 382
8600 LaSalle Rd.
Baltimore, MD 21204
(410) 296-0232 (voice)
(800) 222-3123 (voice)
(410) 321-5069 (fax)

Parent Advocacy Coalition for
Educational Rights (PACER)
Center
4826 Chicago Ave., S
Minneapolis, MN 55417
(612) 827-2966 (voice)

President's Committee on
Mental Retardation
330 Independence Ave., SW,
   Room 5325
Washington, DC 20201
(202) 619-0634 (voice)

Schizophrenia Research Branch,
Division of Clinical and Treatment
   Research,
National Institute of Mental
   Health
5600 Fishers Ln.
Parklawn Building, Room 18C14
Rockville, MD 20857
(301) 443-4707 (voice)
(301) 443-6000 (fax)

Social Security Administration
Office of Communications
W. High Rise Building.
6401 Security Blvd., Room 4200
Baltimore, MD 21235
(410) 965-1720 (voice)
(800) 772-1213 (voice)

Tourette Syndrome Association
42-40 Bell Blvd.
Bayside, NY 11361
(718) 224-2999 (voice)
(800) 237-0717 (voice)
(718) 279-9596 (fax)

NUMBERS OF CHILDREN AFFECTED BY BEHAVIORAL, LEARNING, AND EMOTIONAL DISORDERS*

- One in every five children and adolescents has a mental health problem at any given time.

- One in every twenty young people is affected by a serious emotional disturbance at any given time.

- Eight to ten in every one hundred children and adolescents are affected by an anxiety disorder (phobia, generalized anxiety disorder, panic disorder, obsessive-compulsive disorder, post-traumatic stress disorder).

- One in every one hundred adults is affected with bipolar disorder (symptoms often begin in the teenage years).

- Five in every one hundred children are identified with a learning disorder in the public school system.

- Five in every one hundred children have attention deficit hyperactivity disorder.

- Four to ten in every one hundred children and adolescents have conduct disorder.

- One in every one hundred to two hundred adolescent girls has anorexia.

- One to three in every one hundred young people has bulimia nervosa.

- Seven to fourteen in every ten thousand children have autism spectrum disorder.

- Three in every one thousand adolescents have schizophrenia.

*Statistics from U.S. Department of Health and Human Services, Center for Mental Health Services

RECOMMENDED READING

Alexander-Roberts, Colleen. *The ADHD Parenting Handbook*. Dallas: Taylor Publishing Company, 1994.

———. *ADHD and Teens: A Parent's Guide to Making It through the Tough Years*. Dallas: Taylor Publishing Company, 1995.

Comings, David E. *Tourette Syndrome and Human Behavior*. Duarte, CA: Hope Press, 1990.

Farber, Adele and Elaine Mazlish. *How to Talk So Kids Will Listen and Listen So Kids Will Talk*. New York: Rawson, Wade Publishers, 1980.

Griffin, Mary, and Carol Felsenthal. *A Cry for Help*. Garden City, NY: Doubleday, 1983.

Hearle, Tracy, ed. *Children with Tourette Syndrome: A Parents' Guide*. Rockville, MD: Woodbine House, 1992.

Ingersoll, Barbara D., and Sam Goldstein. *Lonely, Sad and Angry: A Parent's Guide to Depression in Children and Adolescents*. New York: Doubleday, 1995.

Kelly, Dorothy A. *Central Auditory Processing Disorder: Strategies for Use in Children and Adolescents*. Tucson, AZ: the Psychological Corporation, 1995.

Kerns, Lawrence, L., with Adrienne B. Lieberman. *Helping Your Depressed Child*. (Rocklin, CA: Prima Publishing, 1993.

Levine, Mel. *Keeping a Head in School*. Cambridge, MA: Educators Publishing Service, 1991.

Looney, John G., ed. *Chronic Mental Illness in Children and Adolescents*. Washington, DC: American Psychiatric Press, 1988.

Love, Harold D. *Behavior Disorders in Children: A Book for Parents*. Springfield, IL: Thomas, 1987.

McKnew, Donald H., and Leon Cytryn. *Growing up Sad: Childhood Depression and Its Treatment*. New York: WW. Norton, 1996.

Oster, Gerald D., and Sarah S. Montgomery. *Helping Your Depressed Teenager: A Guide for Parents and Caregivers*. New York: John Wiley & Sons, 1995.

Rapoport, Judith. *The Boy Who Couldn't Stop Washing: The Experience and Treatment of Obsessive-Compulsive Disorder*. New York: Dutton, 1989.

Sills, Judith. *Excess Baggage: Getting out of Your Own Way*. New York: Penguin, 1993.

Silver, Larry B. *The Misunderstood Child: A Guide for Parents of Children with Learning Disabilities*, rev. ed. Blue Ridge Summit, PA: TAB, 1992.

Turecki, Stanley. *The Difficult Child*. New York: Bantam, 1985.

———. *The Emotional Problems of Normal Children*. New York: Bantam, 1994.

Vail, Priscilla. *Smart Kids with School Problems: Things to Know and Ways to Help*. New York: New American Library, 1987.

———. *Learning Styles: Food for Thought and 130 Practical Tips*. Rosemont, NJ: Modern Learning Press, 1993.

Windell, James. *Discipline: A Sourcebook of 50 Failsafe Techniques for Parents*. New York: Collier, 1991.

Wing, Lorna. *Autistic Children: A Guide for Parents and Professionals*. New York: Brunner/Mazel, 1985.

Youngs, Bettie B. *How to Develop Self-Esteem in Your Child:*

Six Vital Ingredients. New York: Fawcett Columbine, 1991.

GLOSSARY

Acute illness An illness of short duration, marked by rapid onset and severe symptoms.

Addiction Most often used to refer to physical dependence on a substance such as alcohol or other drugs. Deprived of the drug they're addicted to, addicts may suffer withdrawal symptoms.

Adjustment disorder This is a disorder in which the individual is unable to adjust to difficult and stressful life events, such as a family crisis, a divorce, or a severely changed economic situation. Results in impaired functioning, usually in all areas of life. Emotional and behavioral reactions are often out of proportion to provoking circumstance. As defined, these symptoms last less than six months.

Affect A term often used by mental health professionals to refer to the type and degree of emotion than an individual displays. A lack of emotional expression is called "blunted affect," and often accompanies depression. To show "appropriate affect" means to display emotions that fit the situation at hand. "Inappropriate affect" indicates an abnormal emotional response, like laughing when presented with tragedy.

Affective disorder A disorder of mood, characterized by mood disturbance. Depression and bipolar disorder are examples.

Amphetamines A class of drugs that are central nervous system stimulants. Used with great success in the treatment of ADHD/ADD. For individuals who don't have these disorders, they can be abused.

Anorexia nervosa Characterized by a fear of obesity, this is an eating disorder that leads to a distorted body image (seeing oneself as fat when actually seriously underweight) and often bizarre dietary restrictions.

Antianxiety drugs Medication taken by prescription to lessen symptoms of anxiety. Have been referred to as tranquilizers.

Antidepressant drugs Medication taken by prescription to treat depression. Tricyclics and SSRIs (serotonin specific reuptake inhibitors—Prozac, Zoloft, Paxil) are examples of two main classes.

Antipsychotic drugs Medication taken by prescription to treat psychosis or psychotic-like behaviors. Also called *neuroleptic drugs* and *major tranquilizers*.

Antisocial personality disorder The adult equivalent of adolescent conduct disorder; the person must be over eighteen years old to be diagnosed. A disorder marked by the individual's inability to abide by societal rules, a lack of concern for the feelings, needs, or rights of others. Such a person also is referred to by some as a psychopath or sociopath.

Anxiety Classically described as a feeling of apprehension, as if something terrible were about to happen, a sense of impending doom. Often associated with unpleasant body sensations such as rapid heartbeat, sweating, shortness of breath, palpitations, abdominal distress, and chest pain. Sometimes patients believe they're experiencing a heart attack.

Anxiety disorder A psychiatric disorder in which anxiety is the main symptom. Obsessive-compulsive disorder and phobias are anxiety disorders often seen in children, as is post-traumatic stress disorder, especially following moderate to severe abuse. Panic attacks are also an anxiety disorder.

Assessment A professional review of a child's and family's needs performed by a therapist when the family first seeks services. The assessment includes a review of the child's physical and mental health, intelligence, school performance, family situation, and behavior. It identifies areas of concern and strength, as well as areas of potential growth.

Attention deficit disorder (ADD) Considered by many in the field to be a subset of attention deficit hyperactivity disorder, with the lack of hyperactivity as the primary difference.

Attention deficit hyperactivity disorder (ADHD) A disorder that starts in childhood. Contrary to popular belief, it isn't actually a deficit in attention, but rather an inability to focus one's attention at will and to maintain that focus. Impulsive behavior and increased motor activity are seen. Often treated with central nervous system stimulants with high success. A complete treatment regimen demands evaluation for comorbidities such as depression, oppositional defiant disorder, conduct disorder, and others.

Autism A syndrome first appearing in childhood. Prominent symptoms are self-absorption and a seeming lack of need for stimulation from others or the outside world. Odd behaviors such as constant rocking motions, along with severely impaired communications skills mark these children as different from their age peers. Also known as pervasive developmental disorder (PDD). Sometimes incorrectly referred to as childhood schizophrenia.

Autonomic nervous system Controls involuntary body functions that are carried on automatically without thought, such as breathing, heartbeat, digestion, et cetera. It is further divided into the sympathetic nervous system and the parasympathetic nervous system.

Avoidant personality disorder A disorder in which the individual is often overly sensitive to rejection, experiencing profound discomfort in situations involving social contact. Those with the disorder usually reduce social contact to minimal levels over time.

Bed-wetting *See* enuresis.

Behavioral therapy A short-term psychotherapy aimed at changing specific behaviors.

Biofeedback A type of relaxation training that uses instrumentation to measure heart rate and muscle tension while the person practices deep relaxation techniques.

Bipolar disorder Formerly called manic-depression. An affective disorder in which periods of depression alternate with manic periods of high energy, grandiosity, and excitement.

Borderline personality disorder A disorder with rapidly changing mood, very unstable personal relationships, and a lack of identity.

Bruxism Grinding of the teeth, most frequently occurring during sleep.

Bulimia nervosa An eating disorder in which binge eating is followed by purging by vomiting or heavy laxative use, or by both.

Character Sometimes called *personality*, it is the collection of an individual's unique emotional, behavioral, and intellectual patterns. It is affected by environment and is stable over time.

Chronic illness An illness of long duration. Contrast to *acute illness*.

Codependent A colloquial term, it has achieved great use among mental health professionals. Used to describe the relationship between two people who share a maladaptive relationship involving addiction to people (frequently, each other), places, or things (often, drugs or alcohol).

Cognition The so-called higher functions of the mind: judgment, reasoning, intuition, perception, and memory.

Cognitive development The process over time as a child develops his thinking and problem-solving skills.

Cognitive therapy A short-term therapy that focuses on replacing poor coping skills with more effective ones by changing distorted thinking that causes or contributes to problems.

Compliance Effectively following a physician's recommendations for the use of medications and any other recommended therapeutic modalities.

Compulsion A powerful need to perform an act or to perform an act in a certain, highly specific way, over and over again. Failure to perform can lead to great anxiety.

Conditioning Changing behavior through the use of learning. Using a stimulus to evoke a response is called *classical*, or *Pavlovian*, conditioning. American psychologist B. F. Skinner demonstrated operant conditioning in which reward or punishment is used to change behavior.

Conduct disorder Generally diagnosed in children under age fifteen, it is the adolescent analogue of the adult diagnosis of antisocial personality disorder. Affected children often cheat, steal, lie, fight, and generally disregard the rights of others.

Continuum of care A progression of services that a child moves through as needed. Often, portions of different services are combined to better serve the needs of the child at that time.

Crisis intervention A type of therapy used in intervention of psychiatric crisis. Aimed at restoring coping ability and ending the acute crisis.

Crisis residential treatment services Short-term, around-the-clock help provided during a crisis in a nonhospital setting. Example: If a child becomes aggressive and uncontrollable, the parent can have the child temporarily placed in a *crisis residential treatment service*. The purpose of this is to stabilize the child's condition, while protecting him from harming himself or others. In that controlled setting, a more rational determination of the next appropriate step is possible, while avoiding inpatient hospitalization unless absolutely necessary.

CT scan An imaging device used to examine the interior of the body. Used in psychiatry to detect brain abnormalities related to some psychiatric disorders.

Cyclothymia A milder form of bipolar disorder; mood swings are the most salient characteristic.

Day hospital An alternative to the choice of outpatient care versus hospitalization. Psychiatric hospital care in which the patient is admitted during the day but is released to return home at night.

Day treatment Day treatment usually includes most or all of the following: special education, counseling, vocational training, skill building, crisis intervention, recreational therapy, and parent training. It generally lasts at least four hours a day, but can last longer. Day treatment programs are often a part of mental health, educational, or recreational organizations.

Defense mechanism An unconscious and automatic response to a perceived threat. Any situation that evokes anxiety or fear can serve as a trigger. Contrast to a conscious, intentional defense of one's position.

Delirium Acute mental confusion and disorientation, with an inability to focus on and deal effectively with the immediate environment or to process information.

Delirium tremens Mental and physical state sometimes suffered by alcoholics deprived of alcohol. The individual is disoriented, can have hallucinations, often has the "shakes."

Delusion Frequently occurs in schizophrenia. Delusions are false beliefs held as true by the individual, even in the face of incontrovertible proof to the contrary. A person can be delusional without having schizophrenia.

Dementia Generally refers to a loss of mental capacity, usually most notable in loss of memory and intellectual ability. Most often is accompanied by changes in personality and behavior. Some dementias are reversible medically, but some, like Alzheimer's dementia, are not.

Denial A type of defense mechanism in which painful realizations or truths are unconsciously prevented from reaching conscious awareness.

Dependent personality disorder A disorder characterized by poor self-esteem, a lack of both confidence and the ability to make sound decisions quickly. Person is often self-denigrating in thought, speech, and act.

Depression One of the primary affective disorders. Characterized by poor and unhappy mood. Often noted are loss of interest in activities/things that have been favored, changes in sleep and appetite, a sense of fatigue/malaise, feelings of worthlessness and despair, and thoughts of suicide or suicide attempts. Depression can range from the low-intensity but chronic dysthymia to the acute and severe major depression.

Developmental disability Sometimes still referred to as *mental retardation*. A failure in development of age-appropriate cognitive and intellectual capacity.

DNA (deoxyribonucleic acid) Found in each cell of our body, it is the complex protein that carries our individual genetic "blueprint."

Down syndrome A congenital type of mental retardation. This genetic problem is also expressed in a characteristic appearance, particularly in facial features. Children with Down syndrome have an extremely high incidence of serious physical anomalies, particularly cardiac problems.

Drug holiday The temporary discontinuance of one or more of an individual's medications. Drug holidays are used in reevaluation of one's need for a specific drug to allow troublesome side effects to subside, or to prevent or minimize potential long-term, deleterious effects.

DSM-IV (Diagnostic and Statistical Manual of Mental Disorders, Fourth Edition) A highly referred-to manual of mental health problems developed and published by the American Psychiatric Association. This reference book is used by psychiatrists, psychologists, social workers, and other mental health professionals to diagnose mental health problems.

Dyslexia A learning disorder related to language-processing difficulties, specifically reading. In the past, it was most commonly associated with letter reversal when reading. Children with dyslexia often have difficulty associating letters of the alphabet with their assigned sounds. Once called developmental reading disorder, it is now known simply as *reading disorder*.

Early intervention A process of recognizing early warning signs that a child is at risk for developing mental health problems. Intervening quickly may well reduce the extent of illness that develops and prevent more serious difficulties.

Eating disorder Any disorder in which a disturbance in eating behavior is the primary feature. Anorexia nervosa and bulimia nervosa are examples.

Electroconvulsive therapy (ECT) A therapy using electric currents, used primarily to treat depression; also known as shock therapy.

Electroencephalograph (EEG) An instrument used to detect and record brain wave activity.

Emergency and crisis services Services that are available twenty-four hours a day, seven days a week, to assist with a mental health emergency. Examples of such services: crisis hotlines, crisis counseling, crisis residential treatment services, and crisis outreach teams.

Empathy The ability to feel the emotions and experience of others; empathy helps us understand one another.

Enuresis Involuntary release of urine; associated with bed-wetting.

Family therapy Therapy predicated on the belief that each family member affects the others—a systems approach. The family system, not just a member, is treated.

Flooding A behavioral therapy variant that exposes patients to the object of their fear over and over again to desensitize them; used to treat phobias.

Gene The basic unit of heredity. Physical appearance, size—all physical traits—are "coded" by genes. There is mounting evidence that predisposition to an emotional disorder—or having the disorder itself—is also coded genetically.

Generalized anxiety disorder (GAD) An anxiety disorder that is focused on free-floating anxiety, that is, an anxiety unattached to circumstances or situations. The person is always anxious, not just in certain circumstances.

Group therapy A therapeutic environment with two or more clients and the therapist. "Group dynamics," how the individual members of the group interact with each other and the group as a whole, can be valuable and instructive to the therapist in helping each member and in helping each member help the others.

Halfway house Term often used to describe an environment useful to recently discharged psychiatric patients in making the transition from the hospital environment to the world at large.

Hallucination A perception that seems real to the person experiencing it, but that has no basis in reality. May involve any of the five senses, but usually is either aural or visual.

Home-based services Help provided in the home, either for a defined time or for as long as necessary to effectively deal with a mental health problem. Services may include counseling, parent training, and work with other family members as well as the child. The goal is to prevent the child from needing to be removed from the home.

Hyperactivity A state of high physical activity, seen frequently in many young children from time to time; seen as a regular feature in attention deficit hyperactivity disorder.

Hypomania A clinical state almost identical to mania, except that the person is not as excitable nor as likely to be as grandiose. A state of heightened awareness and arousal.

Identity An individual's sense of self based on physical and emotional characteristics and on how he perceives those characteristics.

Inpatient hospitalization Mental health treatment in a hospital setting twenty-four hours a day. Inpatient hospitalization is used for short-term treatment when a child is in crisis and possibly a danger to self or others and for diagnosis and treatment when outpatient services are either not possible or would be inappropriate.

Inpatient treatment *See* inpatient hospitalization.

Insight Having an understanding of the unconscious motivations of action; a psychoanalytic term.

Major depression A period of very depressed mood, with loss of interest and pleasure in regular pursuits, lasting at least two weeks. Often accompanied with many of the following: sleep disturbances, appetite changes, poor concentration, reduced self-image, lack of energy. Person may express guilt or have suicidal ideation. Is often recurrent.

Mania A mood disorder expressed by heightened activity, agitation, and usually, euphoria. *See* manic-depression, bipolar disorder.

Manic-depression, manic-depressive disorder *See* bipolar disorder.

Mental disorders *See* mental health problems.

Mental health Refers to how people think, feel, and act when faced with life's situations. It reflects how people see themselves, their lives, and the others who share their lives. It evaluates how people handle the challenges and the problems of their lives. This includes how well they handle stress, relating to other people, and decision making.

Mental health problems Mental health problems range in severity from minor inconvenience through modest difficulty to severe and disabling illness; they are very real. As with any other health problem, they are deserving of prompt diagnosis and effective treatment.

Mental illness This term is often used to refer to the more severe mental health problems.

Mental retardation *See* developmental disability.

Mental status examination A method of evaluating an individual's mental function; may be formal or informal testing.

Minimal brain disorder Former name for ADD/ADHD. Now used to describe minor neurological deficits that influence both learning and movement.

MMPI, MMPI-2 Minnesota Multiphasic Personality Index and second edition. Psychological test used to assess personality traits and styles.

Modeling The process of learning behavior by basing one's own on that of another perceived to be more successful.

Mood An individual's most predominant internal emotional experience; understood as opposed to affect, which is the outward demonstration of emotional feelings.

Mood disorder Literally, a disturbance in mood. Both bipolar disorder and major depression are mood disorders.

Multidisciplinary treatment team In psychiatric environments, treatment of the patient by physicians, social workers, psychologists, nurses, and others as needed to meet the therapeutic needs of the patient.

Mutism Name given to a state in which a patient doesn't speak. May be psychologically or organically determined.

Neurobiological disorder A term used to describe a group of brain disorders or mental illnesses that cause disturbances in thinking, feeling, or relating, resulting in a significantly diminished capacity for coping with the ordinary demands of everyday life.

Neuroleptic drug *See* antipsychotic drug.

Neurologist, neurology Medical specialist who treats diseases of the nervous system; medical specialty field focusing on diseases of the nervous system.

Neurotransmitters Chemical messengers that facilitate communication in the nervous system. Too much or too little of some of these critical messengers can result in psychiatric difficulties.

Night terror The panic-like fear experienced while dreaming; occurs primarily in children.

Nocturnal Occurring at night. For example, "nocturnal sleep" refers to sleep that occurs at night.

Noncompliance Not following a doctor's recommended treatment plan; for example, not taking medications or eating as directed.

Obsession Constantly recurring thought not under control of the individual. May be seen as pleasant, but most often is unpleasant and stressful. Often leads to compulsion.

Obsessive-compulsive disorder A disorder in which certain patterns of thought and behavior become established as major preoccupations. Symptoms may become extremely stressful and seriously compromise the individual's ability to function.

Operant conditioning *See* conditioning.

Oppositional defiant disorder A childhood conduct-specific disorder.

Children who have this disorder are often angry, resentful, and argumentative.

Organic disease Disease of a physical origin.

Outpatient care Care and treatment taking place while the patient resides outside the hospital (no overnight stay).

Panic Severe anxiety, often with terror-like features.

Panic attack An episode of extreme anxiety; physical symptoms frequently seen are chest pain, nausea, sweating, hyperventilation; individual may fear she will die.

Paranoia A mental disorder or syndrome in which the individual has delusions of persecution.

Pathological Descriptive of, or pertaining to, disease.

Pavlov, Ivan (1849-1936) A Russian physiologist who demonstrated the concept of classical conditioning, sometimes referred to as *Pavlovian* conditioning.

Personality The unique collection of emotions, behaviors, and thoughts that determines who a person is.

Pervasive developmental disorder (PDD) *See* autism.

Pharmacotherapy The treatment of disease with pharmacological agents such as medications.

Phobia An irrational, persistent fear that compels one to avoid whatever (person, object, situation) evokes the fear.

Physiology The study of biological function and the operational process of life.

Pica A type of eating disorder in which nonfood items are eaten.

Plan of care A treatment plan designed for each child or family. The therapist or other professional develops the plan with the parents (or family, in family therapy). The plan identifies the child's and family's strengths and needs. It establishes goals and details appropriate treatment and services to meet those needs.

Play therapy A therapy using dolls, cutouts, and drawings to elicit otherwise hard-to-retrieve information from children; also used to provide instruction and therapy to children.

Posttraumatic stress disorder (PTSD) Syndrome that can develop after a severely traumatic experience. Can occur at any age. The traumatic event is often reexperienced through memories and nightmares.

Psychiatrist A physician who has specialized training in the treatment of mental disorders, and who is licensed to prescribe medication for their treatment.

Psychiatry The branch of medicine that focuses on mental disorders.

Psychoanalysis A form of psychotherapy. Established by Sigmund Freud, it looks to unconscious motivations and conflicts to explain behavior and to effect change.

Psychodynamic psychotherapy A form of psychotherapy derived from psychoanalysis. It seeks to change behavior and feelings by discovering and understanding unconscious conflicts and motivations, many of which stem from childhood experiences.

Psychologist A practitioner in psychology; usually holds a Ph.D.

Psychomotor agitation Increased physical activity due to mental upset, unrest, or agitation.

Psychomotor retardation Decreased mental and physical activity, due to mental or emotional status.

Psychopharmacology The study of treating mental illness with medications.

Psychosis Any mental state in which a person's contact with reality is substantially impaired, usually by symptoms of delusion, hallucination, and strange behaviors and beliefs. The psychosis may be acute and temporary or chronic and lifelong.

Psychosocial Having to do with both psychological and sociological factors.

Psychosomatic illness A physical illness that is the result of psychological factors.

Psychotherapist A practitioner of psychotherapy.

Psychotherapy The treatment of psychological disorders that uses so-called talk therapy to relieve symptoms and achieve behavioral change and self-growth.

Psychotic Pertaining to psychosis; one who exhibits symptoms of psychosis.

Psychotropic drug A drug or medication that modifies the function of the mind.

Reality therapy A technique of psychotherapy used to help confused individuals reorient to reality.

Recreational drug A drug used for pleasurable effects without regard to medicinal need or purpose.

Repression The unconscious blocking of painful or threatening experiences from memory; considered a defense mechanism.

Residential treatment centers These facilities provide treatment twenty-four hours a day. Children with serious emotional disturbances can reside there and receive constant supervision and care. Treatment includes individual, group, and behavior therapy; special education; medical services; recreation therapy; and, most often, family therapy. Residential treatment is usually more long term than inpatient hospitalization, often being set up to coincide with school semesters. May also be called *therapeutic group homes*.

Respite care Taking care of any child can sometimes be a strain; continuously taking care of a child with a serious emotional disturbance can put the mental and physical health of parents at serious risk. Respite care provides a needed break for those parents. Sometimes provided in the home; usually the parents get to leave for several hours, or even a day or two. Trained parents or counselors take care of the child while the parents are gone.

Schizophrenia A severe, chronic disturbance of mood, thought, and perception. A form of psychosis, it is frequently associated with delusions and hallucinations.

Sedative hypnotics Medications used to reduce anxiety or to induce sleep.

Serious emotional disturbances Disorders in children and adolescents that severely disrupt daily functioning in the home, school, or community. May include depression, anxiety, conduct, and eating disorders.

Serotonin A neurotransmitter, abnormal levels of which (either too much or too little) can induce mood and behavior changes; believed to be important to the inducement or relief of depression.

Shock therapy *See* electroconvulsive therapy.

Side effect Any effect of a medication other than the intended therapeutic effect.

Somatic Pertaining to bodily function; physical.

Stereotypy, stereotypical behavior Mechanical or rote repetition of words or physical movements and behaviors. Often seen in autism and schizophrenia.

Substance abuse Habitual use of any substance resulting in harm to the individual; those with substance abuse are reluctant to stop using, even when aware of the harmful effect.

Sundowning A phenomenon in which individuals with mental disorders act relatively normal during the daytime, but exhibit bizarre or unusual behaviors at night.

Support group A self-help group consisting of members with similar problems and goals.

Supportive therapy A type of psychotherapy that focuses on restoring coping mechanisms and relieving symptoms.

Suppression Another defense mechanism; here, disturbing thoughts or emotions are consciously put from the mind; contrast to *repression.*

Sympathetic nervous system Part of the autonomic nervous system; controls motor nerves and involuntary muscles.

Syndrome A grouping of symptoms that together comprise a specific disorder.

Tardive dyskinesia A side effect of the use of some antipsychotic medications. Sometimes remits with cessation of the medication; sometimes is irreversible. Involves involuntary movements of facial muscles, tongue, mouth, body, or limbs.

Temperament One aspect of personality; an individual's inborn genetic and biological disposition.

Therapeutic alliance A healing relationship that promotes improvement. Developed between a psychotherapist and his client.

Therapist A person who practices therapy.

Tranquilizer A generic term for medications used to relieve anxiety.

Trauma When used in psychiatry, refers to a disturbing event or experience.

Tricyclic antidepressant One class of antidepressant medications, so-called for its three-ringed chemical configuration.

Unconscious A concept promoted by Freud defining a complex set of drives and feelings beyond conscious awareness that motivate behaviors.

BIBLIOGRAPHY

Adamec, Christine. *How to Live with a Mentally Ill Person.* New York: John Wiley & Sons, 1996.

Alexander-Roberts, Colleen. *The ADHD Parenting Handbook: Practical Advice for Parents from Parents.* Dallas: Taylor Publishing Company, 1994.

————. *ADHD and Teens: A Parent's Guide to Making It through the Tough Years.* Dallas: Taylor Publishing Company, 1995.

American Psychiatric Association. *Diagnosis and Statistical Manual of Mental Disorders, Fourth Edition.* Washington, DC: American Psychiatric Association, 1994.

Bell, Tammy L. "Dysfunctional Parenting Styles." *Addiction and Recovery* (January-February 1992), vol. 12, no. 1, 12(3).

Bower, Bruce. "Troubling Tally of Kids' Mental Disorders." *Science News* (December 24, 1988), vol. 134, no. 26-27, 405(1).

Campbell, Thomas L., and Joan M. Patterson. "The Effectiveness of Family Interventions in the Treatment of Physical Illness." *The Journal of Marital and Family Therapy* (October 1995), vol. 21, no. 4, 545(39).

"Children of Parents with Mental Illness." American Academy of Child and Adolescent Psychiatry (May 6, 1996), no. 39, Facts for Family series.

de Wilde, Erik J., et al. "The Relationship between Adolescent Suicidal Behavior and Life Events in Childhood and Adolescence." *American Journal of Psychiatry* (January 1992), vol. 1149, no. 1, 45(7).

Deal, James E., Charles F. Halverson, and Karen S. Wampler. "Parental Agreement on Child-Rearing Orientations: Relations to Parental, Marital, Family, and Child Characteristics." *Child Development* (1989), vol. 60, 1025-1034.

Doneberg, Geri, and Bruce L. Baker. "The Impact of Young Children with Externalizing Behaviors on their Families." *Journal of Abnormal Child Psychology* (April 1993), vol. 21, no. 2, 179(20).

Hadderman, Margaret. "Learning Disabilities." *ERIC Digest*, no. 407. Revised, 1986.

Hamm, John. "Intensive Day Treatment Provides an Alternative to Residential Care." *Children Today* (September-October 1989), vol. 18, no. 5, 11(5).

"Learning Disabilities: Decade of the Brain." National Institute of Mental Health, NIMH publication no. 93-3611.

McFarlane, William R. "Families in the Treatment of Psychotic Disorders." *Harvard Mental Health Letter* (October 1995), vol. 12, no. 4, 4(3).

Messer, Stephen C., and Deborah C. Beidel. "Psychosocial Correlates of Childhood Anxiety Disorders." *Journal of the American Academy of Child and Adolescent Psychiatry* (September 1994), vol. 33, no. 7, 975(9).

Rapoport, J. L. *Obsessive-Compulsive Disorder in Children and Adolescents.* Washington, DC: American Psychiatric Press, 1989.

Rowe, David C. *The Limits of Family Influence: Genes, Experience, and Behavior.* New York: Guilford Press, 1994.

Smollar, Jacqueline, and Larry Condelli. "Residential Placement of Youth: Pathways, Alternatives, and Unresolved Issues." *Children Today* (November-December 1990), vol. 19, no. 6, 4(5).

Index

A

Absenteeism from school, 33, 120
Abuse of children, 138–139
and aggression, 152
Acceptance of children by parents, 212–213
ADHD. *See* Attention deficit hyperactivity disorder (ADHD)
Adolescents. *See* Teenagers
Adoption, 141–142
Age-appropriateness of behavior, 5, 6–7
Aggression
and abused children, 152
alternatives to, 152
in children, 30, 150–154
in conduct disorder, 68
dealing with, 152–153
and gender, 151–152
genetic predisposition to, 151
in preschoolers, 31
preventing, 153–154
seriousness of, 39
Agoraphobia, 95
Alcoholism. *See also* Substance abuse
and child abuse, 139
and heredity, 20–21
of parent, 140–141
American Academy of Child and Adolescent Psychiatry, 140–141, 159
Anger in children, 150–154
Anhedonia, 88–89
Anorexia nervosa, 98–100, 222
comorbidity with bipolar disorder, 91
Anxiety, 30, 145–146
and desensitization, 184–185
medication for, 145–146
signs of, 145
Anxiety disorders, 93–98, 222
comorbidity with separation anxiety disorder, 119

frequency of, 16
signs and symptoms of, 94
Aphasia, developmental, 107
Appointment with mental health professional
fees for, 162
first, 166–169
calling for, 161–162
conclusion of, 167–168
follow up on, 168–169
preparing for, 162–166
records useful at, 163–165
Archives of General Psychiatry, 17–18
Articulation problems, 58. *See also* Communication disorders
Asperger's disorder (Asperger's syndrome), 49, 51–52
comorbidity with oppositional defiant disorder (ODD), 67
and obsessive-compulsive disorder (OCD), 96
signs and symptoms, 52
Assertiveness training, 185
Attachment disorder, frequency of, 17
Attention deficit hyperactivity disorder (ADHD), 15, 63–66, 114–119, 204, 222
and bipolar disorder, 91, 93
comorbidity with learning disorders, 111–112
comorbidity with obsessive-compulsive disorder (OCD), 96
comorbidity with oppositional defiant disorder (ODD), 67
conditions with symptoms similar to, 117
diagnosing, 116–117
distractibility of children with, 114–116
duration of, 29–30
frequency of, 16, 17
and heredity, 16, 187, 188

and humiliation, 188
medication for, 117–118, 186–187
signs and symptoms of, 64–66
and Tourette's disorder, 72
traits of, 63
treatment of, 117–119
Autism, 49–51, 222
comorbidity with obsessive-compulsive disorder (OCD), 96
frequency of, 17
signs and symptoms of, 50–51

B

Baggage, excess, from own childhood, 201, 203, 205–208
Beck, Aaron, 185
Behavior
difference between normal and problematic, 5
indicating need for therapy, 11–13
parents' view of children's, 7–10
temporary, 11
Behavioral disorders. *See also specific disorders*
frequency of, 4, 222
importance of treatment of, 4–5
multifactorial nature of, 18–19, 26
significance of, for children, 79
sources of information on, 222
Behavioral problems in children with learning disorders, 113–114
Behavioral rehearsal, 185
Behavioral therapies, 183–185
Behavior modification, 121–122
Bereavement psychotherapy, 132